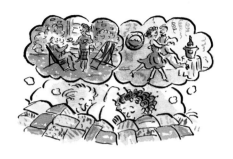

HEALTH AND HEALING
THE NATURAL WAY

HOLDING BACK
THE CLOCK

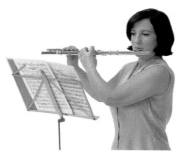

HEALTH AND HEALING
THE NATURAL WAY

HOLDING BACK THE CLOCK

Reader's Digest

PUBLISHED BY

THE READER'S DIGEST ASSOCIATION, INC.

PLEASANTVILLE, NEW YORK / MONTREAL

A READER'S DIGEST BOOK
produced by
Carroll & Brown Limited, London

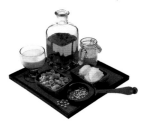

CARROLL & BROWN

Publishing Director Denis Kennedy
Art Director Chrissie Lloyd

Managing Editor Sandra Rigby
Managing Art Editor Tracy Timson

Project Coordinator Laura Price

Editor Denise Alexander
Art Editor Gilda Pacitti

Designers Mercedes Morgan, Vimit Punater

Photographers David Murray, Jules Selmes

Production Karen Kloot, Wendy Rogers

Computer Management John Clifford, Paul Stradling

Printed in the United States of America

Library of Congress Cataloging in Publication Data

Holding Back the Clock
          p. cm. — (Health and healing the natural way)
    Includes index
    ISBN 0-7621-0280-2
        1. Aging—Prevention—Popular works. 2. Longevity—
Popular works. I. Reader's Digest Association. II. Series.
RA776.75 .H65 2000
612.6'8—dc21

                                                    00-020386

The information in this book is for reference only;
it is not intended as a substitute for a doctor's diagnosis and care.
The editors urge anyone with continuing medical problems
or symptoms to consult a doctor.

CONSULTANTS

Professor Tom Kirkwood
*Professor of Biological Gerontology
University of Manchester*

Donald Norfolk DO, FRSH

June Copeman BSc, MSc, MEd, SRD
Leeds Metropolitan University

Debbie Lawrence *Central London YMCA*

Bob Smith MA, BEd (Hons), Cert Ed
Loughborough University

CONTRIBUTORS

Stuart Baker BSc (Hons), PhD
Dr. Michael Denham MD, FRCP
Sharon Freed, BSc, MA
Dr. Lynne Low MBCHB, DA, DFFP, DipGUM
Rick Mattison BSc (Hons), PhD
Angela Newton BA, MA
Donald Norfolk DO, FRSH
Mr. Elliott E Phillip MA, FRCS, FRCOG
Claire Potter; Maria Pufulete; Ian Wood
Dr. Robert Youngson DTM & H, FCOphth

READER'S DIGEST PROJECT STAFF

Series Editor Gayla Visalli
Editorial Director, Health & Medicine Wayne Kalyn
Design Director Barbara Rietschel
Production Technology Manager Douglas A. Croll
Editorial Manager Christine R. Guido
Art Production Coordinator Jennifer R. Tokarski

READER'S DIGEST ILLUSTRATED REFERENCE BOOKS, U.S.

Editor-in-Chief Christopher Cavanagh
Art Director Joan Mazzeo
Operations Manager William J. Cassidy

READER'S DIGEST BOOKS & HOME ENTERTAINMENT, CANADA

Vice President and Editorial Director Deirdre Gilbert
Managing Editor Philomena Rutherford
Art Director John McGuffie

Address any comments about *Holding Back the Clock* to
Editor in Chief, U.S. Illustrated Reference Books,
Pleasantville, NY 10570

HOLDING BACK
THE CLOCK

More and more people today are choosing to take greater responsibility for their own health rather than relying on their doctor to step in with a cure when something goes wrong. It is now recognized that we can influence our health by making certain improvements in lifestyle—eating better, doing more exercise, and taking measures to reduce stress, for example. People are also becoming increasingly aware that there are other healing methods—some new, others ancient—that can help prevent illness or be used as complements to orthodox medicine.

The series *Health and Healing the Natural Way,* which provides clear, comprehensive, straightforward, and encouraging information and advice about methods of improving health, can help you make informed health choices. The series explains the many different natural therapies now available, including aromatherapy, herbalism, acupressure, and a number of others, as well as the circumstances in which they may be of benefit when used in conjunction with conventional medicine.

HOLDING BACK THE CLOCK examines the processes involved in aging and outlines responsible steps you can take at any age to preserve your health, mobility, and a positive mental attitude. Aging does not necessarily lead to illness, loneliness, or depression—many of the problems encountered by the elderly are due to poor lifestyle habits that can easily be changed. In this book you will find strategies for slowing down the aging process, including simple recipes that are rich in vitamins and minerals, an exercise program for people over 50, and mental exercises to help you stay alert and dynamic. It explains how your body ages and describes warning signs of illness to look out for. A healthy diet, regular exercise, and an active mind can literally add years to your life, while sensible use of natural remedies and complementary therapies can help prevent the onset of many ailments or unwelcome effects of aging.

CONTENTS

INTRODUCTION: AGING SUCCESSFULLY 8

 1 THE STAGES OF LIFE

THE AGING PROCESS 16

THEORIES OF AGING 18

The geriatrician 20

FACTORS THAT AFFECT AGING 24

DEALING WITH THE CHANGES
OF AGING 27

An older widower 29

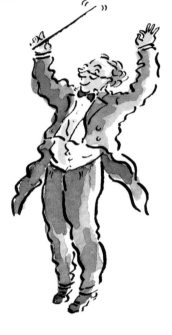

2 A POSITIVE OUTLOOK

CHANGING LIFESTYLES 32

A redundant accountant 34

CHANGING RELATIONSHIPS 36

A marriage under strain 38

Coping with grief 42

KEYS TO HAPPINESS 44

*Expanding your horizons with
new activities 48*

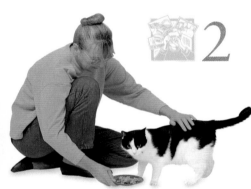

3 FUNCTIONAL HEALTH

MAINTAINING GOOD HEALTH 52

CARDIOVASCULAR SYSTEM 54

RESPIRATORY SYSTEM 58

DIGESTIVE SYSTEM 60

MUSCULOSKELETAL SYSTEM 62

GENITOURINARY SYSTEM 66

THE SENSES 70

ILLNESSES OF THE WHOLE BODY 74

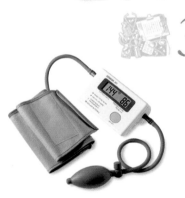

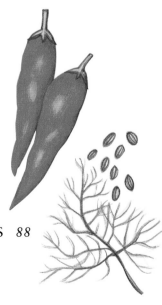

4 YOU ARE WHAT YOU EAT

A HEALTHY DIET 80

ANTIAGING NUTRIENTS 85

DIET AND AGE-RELATED CONDITIONS 88

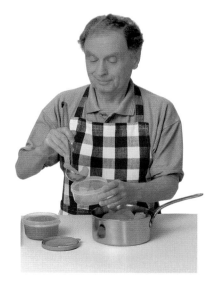

CHANGING EATING HABITS 92
Keeping a productive kitchen garden 94

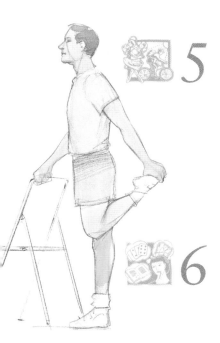

5 STAYING PHYSICALLY ACTIVE
THE IMPORTANCE OF EXERCISE 98
Getting fit with gardening 100
EXERCISE FOR PEOPLE OVER 50 103
Warm-up and flexibility 106
Aqua aerobics 108
Strength exercises 110
OVERCOMING MOBILITY PROBLEMS 112
A retired exerciser 113
Getting fit with line dancing 115

6 AN ACTIVE MIND
HOW AGING AFFECTS YOUR BRAIN 118
The Neurolinguistic programmer 120
A vitamin deficiency 124
EMOTIONS AND AGING 127
Making your bedroom a sleep haven 131
NATURAL THERAPIES
  FOR THE MIND 132

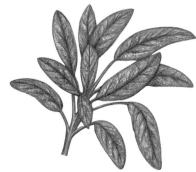

7 LOOKING GOOD,
FEELING GOOD
YOUR PERSONAL STYLE 136
SKIN CARE 141
The dermatologist 144
An insecure woman 148
TEETH AND HAIR 149
FOOT CARE 153
The podiatrist 154

INDEX 157
ACKNOWLEDGMENTS 160

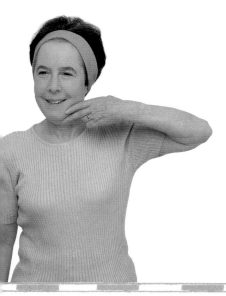

AGING SUCCESSFULLY

With the right attitude, a healthful diet, and an active lifestyle, you can do much to ensure that your later years are both enjoyable and fulfilling.

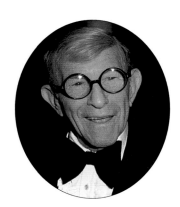

GEORGE BURNS
American comedian George Burns embodied the concept of active retirement. Known as America's favorite geriatric, he remained in the public eye until his death in 1996 at the age of 100.

DIFFERENT VIEWS
During the Renaissance 10 percent of the Venetian population was over 65. Older people were depicted with great dignity in many paintings of the time, as in this detail from a Bellini work.

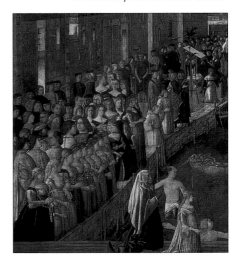

A large portion of the North American population is now older than 60 and the numbers are climbing steadily. In 1999 people over age 60 accounted for nearly 16 percent of the population, and by 2026 the number is expected to climb to 20 percent; people over 85 belong to the fastest growing group in the population today. There are several reasons for this growth. For one, people are living longer. In 1900 life expectancy was about 47 years; by 1999 it was 76 years of age for men and women combined (on average, women live seven to nine years longer than men). Improvements in health technology have contributed to increased life expectancy, partly through eradication or control of many infectious diseases with vaccinations and better hygiene and partly through more effective treatment of illnesses and accidents. People are also having fewer children, so the average age of the population is rising.

Not surprisingly, there is growing concern about the expected burden that such a large number of elderly people will place on society as a whole. However, some of these worries are unfounded. In fact, the elderly are healthier, wealthier, and more secure than they have been for centuries.

There is mounting evidence of the role that diet, exercise, and lifestyle play in reducing the negative effects of aging and preventing many chronic diseases. The assumption that growing older is inexorably connected with debilitating illness is gradually being modified. And there is greater recognition that society can benefit greatly from the vast knowledge and experience of its older population. History provides many examples of people who have participated actively in fields as diverse as the arts, medicine, and law throughout their seventies, eighties, and nineties. Gerontologists, doctors who treat the elderly and observe the effects of aging, believe that current negative impressions of the older population must be rejected before they become a self-fulfilling prophecy.

WHY DO WE AGE?

The maximum life span of humans is believed to be about 120 years, although very few people actually reach this age. Gerontologists are trying to discover the reasons that more people do not attain this maximum and are investigating how our later years can be healthier. Theories about why people age tend to fall into two main categories. The first is that cells deteriorate over time as a result of wear and tear, until they are unable to sustain life. The second is that cells are programmed to die after a certain time span. Most gerontologists believe that a combination of both processes causes humans to age.

Some plant and animal cells appear to be essentially immortal, and scientists have studied these to see if they hold any clues to human aging. The California giant redwood (*Sequoiadendron giganteum*), for example, has a life span of more than 25,000 years, and some seeds discovered in Egyptian tombs have been germinated thousands of years after they were first collected.

Some human cells also seem to bypass the natural process of cell death, but the consequences of this behavior are grave. Cancer cells, for instance, continue to grow and reproduce until they cause irreparable damage to the normal cells around them. During the 1950s in the United States, cells were taken for study from Helen Lack, a woman who was dying of cancer. Her cells, known throughout the scientific community as HeLa cells, are still thriving, reproducing, and growing today—more than 45 years after her death. Clues to the nature of these cells and why they appear to defeat the normal cell life span are being sought by researchers who study aging and the theory of programmed cell death.

THE QUEST FOR LONGEVITY

Gerontology is a modern scientific manifestation of people's fascination with holding back the clock, which has been evident throughout history. As early as 1600 B.C. an Egyptian papyrus described the transformation of an old man into a youth of 20, giving instructions on how to prepare an ointment that it claimed "has been found effective myriad times." There are numerous myths about attempts to gain immortality or cheat death. Orpheus tried to bring his beloved Eurydice back to life; Orion was immortalized as a constellation; and Narcissus was transformed into a flower.

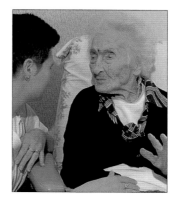

JEANNE CALMENT
When Frenchwoman Jeanne Calment died in 1997 at the age of 122, she was the oldest known person in the world.

HELA CELLS
HeLa cells, pictured below, are kept in laboratories around the world. Because they provide clues about why some cells remain immortal and others age and die, they have been invaluable to researchers.

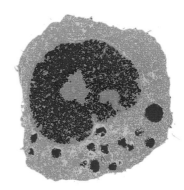

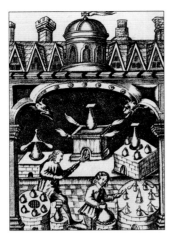

ALCHEMY
Medieval alchemists sought to discover the elixir of life through elaborate but ultimately unsuccessful scientific experiments.

TANSY
The herb tansy has long been associated with immortality. Its name comes from the Greek athanaton, *which means "immortal." In classical mythology tansy was given to the Trojan Ganymede to make him live forever. (We now know that tansy can be toxic; it is generally not recommended for medicinal purposes.)*

Other myths describe ways to restore youth or to find the "fountain of youth," which is also referred to in the Bible, the Koran, ancient Greek and Roman writings, and Hindu writings. Magic water, fruits, precious stones, and many other substances have at one time or another been said to prolong life. In the Middle Ages it was thought that alchemy could be used to produce the "elixir of life." The theme of cheating age has always been popular in Hollywood, with *Shangrila, Cocoon,* and *Indiana Jones and the Last Crusade* being three offerings in the genre.

In the 1800s and 1900s methods for prolonging life became more scientific but no more successful. Some believed that the testicles of humans and animals were the key to longevity. Experiments were carried out on thousands of people, grafting the testicles of animals onto them or injecting them with extracts from animal testicles. At one time even the testicles of dead men were transplanted to healthy males. Needless to say, immortality or rejuvenation did not result. But animal transplants are still being used in the attempt to prolong life. Experiments have also utilized the cells of animal fetuses and sometimes the cells in animal fluids.

In the early 1900s a popular theory evolved that yogurt could extend life. Evidence for this was supposedly seen in the longevity of eastern Europeans who were known to eat yogurt in large amounts. The theory was given further weight by the claims of Elie Metchnikoff, a scientist studying aging. Metchnikoff believed the live bacteria in yogurt would preserve and extend life. Although yogurt with live cultures has many health-giving properties, the claim that it increases longevity has not been proved.

One of the most popular antiaging remedies produced in the 20th century was Gerovital, an anesthetic made from procaine hydrochloride. The makers of Gerovital claimed in the 1950s that it would reverse aging. Sales skyrocketed, but no research has ever proved its effectiveness.

EASTERN CONCEPTS OF AGING

In contrast to Western searches for elixirs of life, Eastern approaches to longevity have tended to embrace holistic health. Taoists, for example, have always believed that eternal youth and immortality can be obtained if one achieves the correct balance of yin and yang energies in the body. Sixth-century Taoist writings explained this theory, and the therapies that evolved to address imbalances in yin and yang energy, such as acupuncture, t'ai chi, and feng shui, form the basis of traditional Chinese lifestyle practices and medicine. Central to Eastern philosophy is the need to exercise, maintain a balanced diet, and preserve a relaxed and calm emotional state. A Taoist adept, Lee Ching-Yuen, who is believed to have lived to an extraordinarily old age, attributed his longevity to three primary rules: take life slowly and calmly; avoid extreme emotions of all kinds; and observe a daily regimen of exercise and deep breathing. In addition, he recommended following a primarily vegetarian diet supplemented by medicinal herbs. Interestingly, this advice is very similar to that given by Western specialists in aging today. They recommend regular exercise to maintain muscle tone and strength; a diet that is not necessarily vegetarian but oriented more toward fruits, vegetables, and whole grains than meat; and the practicing of relaxation techniques to limit the negative effects of stress and anxiety.

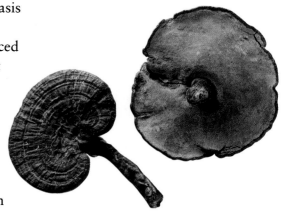

REISHI MUSHROOM
This fungus, dubbed by Taoist scholars the "Mushroom of Deathlessness," is associated with energy and increased longevity. It helps improve circulation and has pain-killing properties. It is also an antioxidant and is said to boost the immune system.

USE IT OR LOSE IT

The best advice for successful aging seems to be to remain active both mentally and physically. Research has shown that at any age the body continues to respond to the demands placed on it. Although some decline in muscle strength occurs over a lifetime, a sedentary lifestyle causes more muscle weakness than the natural effects of aging. Those who exercise regularly retain enough strength to remain independent and mobile. Similarly, science has shown that regular mental stimulation can encourage the growth of dendrites in the brain; these facilitate communication between brain cells and nerves and thus can help compensate for the natural loss of brain cells that occurs throughout life. Activities such as playing chess, completing the crossword in a daily newspaper, or even just keeping up with current affairs can all help maintain an alert and active mind.

USING YOUR MIND
Regularly exercising your mind will help keep you alert and lucid. Playing games such as bridge, in which you have to keep track of what is going on, can improve your memory and mental capacity.

YOUR LIFE IN YOUR HANDS

Two important factors for enjoying old age are cultivation of a positive attitude and brushing aside of any negative stereotypes you may have of older people. If you make up your mind to enjoy life and are proud of your age, your self-esteem will be higher and you will be more likely to retain better health. People of all ages have their highs and lows, and they need a positive attitude to make the most of whatever happens. Ideally, later life should be fulfilling

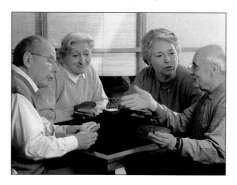

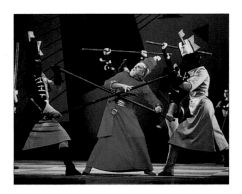

ROBERT HELPMANN
Australian ballet dancer
Robert Helpmann remained
very active throughout his
life. He is seen here (in red)
at age 77 dancing with the
Australian National Ballet
in Checkmate, *which he*
choreographed himself.

SWIMMING
Many older people recognize
that the pursuit of fitness is
an enjoyable and essential
part of life. Regular exercise
can provide huge benefits for
health and well-being.

rather than plagued by illness or loneliness. Overall good health includes mental, emotional, physical, and social well-being. Taking control over each of these aspects will enhance your independence and improve your quality of life. As an individual you can make decisions and take responsibility for yourself. Getting older should not erode this ability. The effect of a positive attitude on physical health and on what you can do should not be underestimated.

HOLDING BACK THE CLOCK

This book aims to provide you with the knowledge you need to make your later years happy and productive. By making the right decisions about your health now, you can greatly improve your chances of enjoying a healthy, active, and satisfying old age.

Chapter 1 explains the theories of aging—including what causes our cells to deteriorate and finally die. Various factors that affect aging, both those you can control or change and those you can't, are also described. Chapter 2 provides an overview of how best to create a positive attitude about your later years. The upheavals of changing relationships, retirement, moving, and taking up new hobbies are all discussed. The changes that your body will undergo with age are described in Chapter 3, along with advice on how to prevent some of those changes or limit the likelihood of developing chronic disease or illness. This chapter also contains guides to important symptoms that warrant seeking medical advice.

Chapters 4 and 5 are about lifestyle. Chapter 4 explains how nutritional needs change as you grow older and gives sound dietary advice on maintaining a healthy body. Recipes are provided to help you make the most of healthy ingredients and include them in your diet every day. Chapter 5 reveals how exercise can not only slow down the effects of aging but actually reverse some of them. The fully illustrated exercise program will enable you to maintain your vitality. Chapter 5 also describes how you can easily incorporate exercise into your daily life.

The effect of aging on the brain and mind is covered in Chapter 6, along with ideas and exercises to stimulate your brain and memory function. The adage "use it or lose it" is especially true when applied to mental acuity. Finally, Chapter 7 looks at how aging affects appearance and what you can do to look your best.

Do you know how to slow the effects of aging?

Many people believe that they simply have to put up with the aches and infirmities of getting older. They expect to become stiff and weak, to forget things, and to lead a sedentary life. These people don't realize that lifestyle choices can be the key to good health throughout life.

Q **DO YOU HAVE LESS ENERGY THAN YOU USED TO?**
It is a common assumption that elderly people have dramatically reduced amounts of energy. Often, however, lower energy levels are simply the result of not doing enough exercise after retirement and spending days in relatively sedentary activities. Try taking a brisk walk every morning, and you will find your energy levels improving. Chapter 5 offers more ideas on exercise.

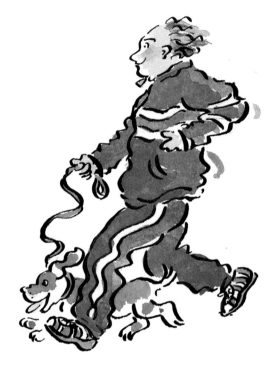

Q **WOULD YOU LIKE TO LEARN A NEW SKILL BUT LACK THE CONFIDENCE?**
It is never too late to learn. After retirement you will have more time to do what you want than perhaps at any other time in your life. It is well worth the effort to join a class or take up a sport or hobby that you wish to try. See Chapter 2.

Q **DO YOU FIND YOURSELF CONSTANTLY FORGETTING WHERE YOU PUT THINGS?**
It is a myth that memory must steadily deteriorate with old age. While we do lose a number of brain cells as we age that are not replaced, and memory does slow down slightly, the brain has the capacity to improve communication between brain cells; it simply requires stimulation. The brain can be exercised and strengthened just like a muscle. Making lists and organizing your thoughts can help to improve your mind power. See Chapter 6.

Q **ARE YOU BOTHERED BY NEW ACHES AND PAINS BUT FEEL THAT THEY ARE TOO TRIVIAL TO CONSULT YOUR DOCTOR ABOUT?**
Aging does not mean that you will inevitably become ill or infirm. If you have a well-balanced diet and exercise regularly, you should remain in relatively good health. If you suffer with aches and pains, see your doctor to determine the cause. This is important not only to rule out serious

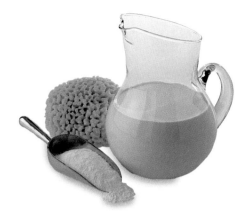

illness but also to find out what the problem is so you can take effective action yourself to relieve the symptoms. See Chapter 3.

Q ARE YOU CONCERNED ABOUT YOUR CHANGING LOOKS?

It can seem alarming when you look in the mirror and see the changes that time has made to your looks. However, growing older does not mean becoming unattractive. Looking healthy and happy is increasingly seen as more important than looking young. A new haircut, flattering clothes, and a healthy, glowing skin can revitalize your appearance and the way you feel about yourself. See Chapter 7.

Q ARE YOU WORRIED THAT RETIREMENT MEANS THE END OF AN ACTIVE LIFE?

Retirement should be regarded as a change rather than an ending. It is a reward that you have worked for. A new door is opening. Chapter 2 has many suggestions for ways in which you can ensure yourself a satisfying retirement and spend your time enjoyably and productively. Retirement may signal the end of paid employment but not the end of your ability to make a valuable contribution to society.

Q ARE YOU AFRAID THAT YOU WILL BE ALONE AND VULNERABLE IN LATER LIFE?

If you are with a partner, the time you have together in old age can be the best of your life. Uninterrupted by children or work, you can enjoy many varied experiences together. Whether you are single or part of a couple, if you make an effort to be sociable, involve yourself in activities, and keep in touch with family and friends, you may be surprised how full your life can be. See Chapter 2.

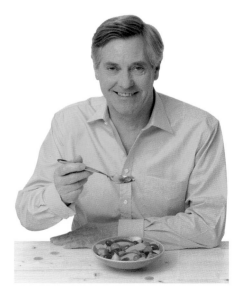

Q ARE YOU CONFUSED BY THEORIES ABOUT TAKING VITAMINS TO BEAT AGING?

Some people believe that taking large doses of antioxidant vitamins and minerals or certain herbs can increase health and longevity. However, there is always a danger of overdosing on supplements because some vitamins and minerals are toxic in large doses and act like drugs in your system. It is better to increase the amount of fruits and vegetables in your diet. With this approach you will also get a more balanced spread of nutrients. See Chapter 4.

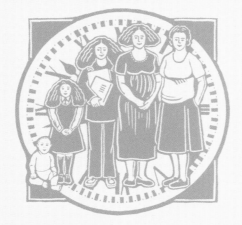

CHAPTER 1

THE STAGES OF LIFE

---

*Why do we age? Why, after we have reached
the height of our physical and mental powers,
do our bodies begin to decline in fitness, strength,
appearance, and often capability? Are these
changes inevitable? The answers to these questions
are still being sought, but we do have some
clues about how to slow the process.*

THE AGING PROCESS

The process of aging is a complex one. Scientists have identified three types of aging that all humans undergo: chronological, biological, and psychological.

THE SEVEN AGES
OF MAN
In his play As You Like
It, *William Shakespeare
described life as
consisting of seven
stages, each with distinct
characteristics. The
modern equivalents of
those stages are described
below. Increasingly,
however, stereotypes are
being challenged; in
particular, negative
concepts of old age are
being rejected.*

Aging is a process that begins the moment we are born. Each body's growth and development are genetically determined, and all of us are subject to biological change. However, much recent research has focused on the significance of such factors as diet and exercise in slowing down aging and maintaining a good quality of life well into old age. But what exactly is involved in the process?

There are two periods of maximal human growth rate. The first, which lasts from birth to age two, is really an extension of the extraordinarily rapid period of fetal growth. The second period starts at puberty and progresses until the early twenties, with all body growth normally complete by age 25. Up to age 30 there is generally progressive improvement and increasing power of both mind and body. After this age some people begin a gradual decline in physical and mental vigor; however, this process is very much dependent on lifestyle. Most people do not experience a noticeable decline until their forties, fifties, or even sixties.

Intellectual and physical capacity often develop at different rates. Commonly during the aging process physical capacity declines while mental capacity continues to increase. Some people's mental capacity reaches its peak during the fifth or sixth decade and then begins to fall off.

While intellectual and physical changes are taking place, we also have to face the psychological demands of the various stages of life; the stresses of these may affect our physical health and the rate at which we age. In each stage there are different challenges, successes, and disappointments to be overcome and enjoyed. In the West we tend to focus on the negative aspects of aging, and for many people later life does bring difficult challenges. However, it is also a time of new freedoms and opportunities.

Babies and toddlers
Early childhood is a time of very rapid growth and an enormous amount of development.

Children
Childhood is a time of extensive learning—physical, intellectual, and emotional.

Adolescents
Adolescence involves growing independence, the forming of strong relationships outside the family, and the development of sexual identity.

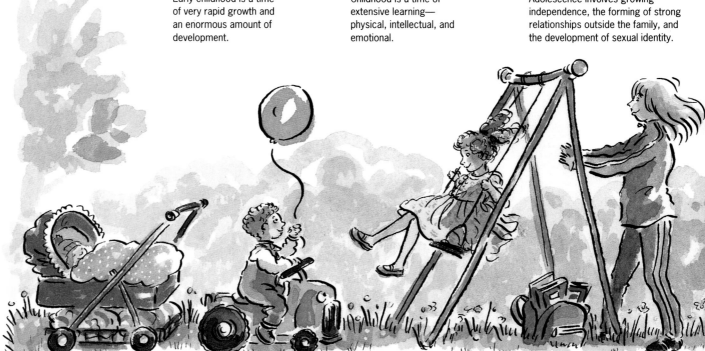

THE MEANING OF AGE

There is a notion that people of a particular age should conform to a certain pattern of behavior. We all think we know what aging looks and feels like. We can identify friends and relatives who we think are "old." This is a subjective view that does not take into account the capacity of the individual to remain physically and mentally able well into old age. Of the three types of aging—chronological, biological, and psychological—only chronological age applies equally to everyone, while biological and psychological age are unique to each individual.

Chronological age is based on the calendar; it refers to the number of years that have passed since you were born. Chronological age tells us very little about how old an individual is because people are very much individuals when it comes to aging. The ageist stereotype predicates that at a certain chronological age, often arbitrarily set at 65, people should retire from paid employment and take up a quieter, more sedentary life. This view is increasingly disputed by many people in society.

Biological age is manifested by all the well-known physical and mental signs of aging. In the stereotype it is assumed that biological age is related to chronological age, but this is not true. Individuals vary greatly in the extent to which they begin to show physical and mental signs of aging. A 70-year-old person who has continued to engage in mentally stimulating activities may be just as mentally capable as a 55-year-old. Similarly, a 65-year-old who has kept physically fit may be able to outrun a 40-year-old who is overweight, who smokes, and who rarely exercises.

Lifestyle is very important in determining biological age. Some scientists are now investigating biomarkers (see page 28). These measurements of the signs of aging can be used to determine biological age. The encouraging thing about these important biomarkers is that some of them are under the control of each individual and can be dramatically improved by the combination of a good diet and sensible exercise.

Psychological age is your own perception of how old you are. We all know the adage "you are as old as you feel," and this is actually true. Those people who continue to be active and do the things they have enjoyed in their younger years are more likely to feel younger. There is also a lot of truth in the saying "use it or lose it." The more stimulation your body gets in the form of exercise and mental activity, the more efficient it will remain, both physically and mentally. Psychological age can also depend to some extent on the attitudes of people you live and work with. Negative and defeatist attitudes can be discouraging and ultimately disabling, while a positive outlook and approach can improve both your physical health and emotional well-being.

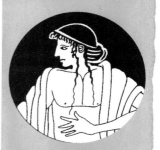

THROUGH THE AGES

Tithonus
The Greek legend of Tithonus is a cautionary tale that demonstrates the importance of health in regard to the quality of life. Tithonus asked the gods to make him immortal but forgot to ask for everlasting youth and vitality. As his body deteriorated, he became disconsolate and prayed to die. The gods turned him into a grasshopper so he could shed his skin every year.

Young adults (twenties and thirties)
Young adulthood sees the development of a career, the forming of long-term relationships, and for many, the start of a family.

Middle agers
Midlife often sees career progression or change, the possible departure of children, and the needs of aging parents to attend to.

Newly retired
This is a time of both positive and negative changes—adjusting to not working and reduced income, having more leisure time, becoming a grandparent, and coping with the illness or death of a spouse or long-time friends.

Elderly
In old age physical and mental abilities may begin to slow down and there may be loss of independence. However, this is also a time of great freedom to enjoy family and friends and pursue leisure interests.

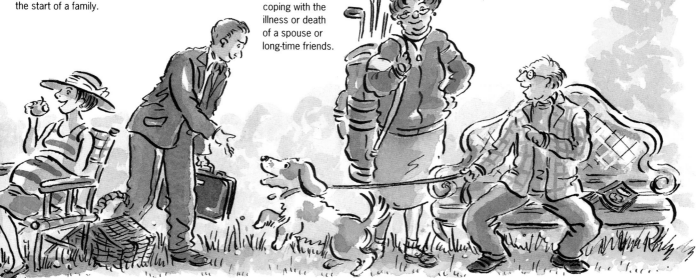

THEORIES OF AGING

There are a number of theories to explain why and how we age. Some of them have contributed significantly to our understanding of how the aging process may be slowed down.

Theories that seek to explain the phenomenon of aging divide into two main categories. One suggests that the body's cells have a predetermined program of aging and death. Another proposes that aging occurs as a result of damage to the body's systems.

The theory of preprogrammed cell death makes sense in evolutionary terms because it is based on the idea that organisms live only long enough to reproduce and care for their young. Immortality and continuing reproduction are incompatible. The earth's environment would not be able to sustain indefinitely prolonged life spans. In other words, without aging and death, the human race could not continue to exist.

Scientists are investigating whether evolution has indeed brought about aging. A few primitive animals, such as reptiles and sharks, do not age. After they reach maturity, they continue to increase in size indefinitely and experience no losses in their normal function. These animals do not live forever, though, because they are still at risk of dying from accidents, disease, and attack from other creatures. Most other animals, however, do undergo aging. It is now known that certain genes determine whether cells reproduce or not, and cell reproduction is essential for life. Programmed cell death organized by genes, in which cells actually kill themselves, is now so well recognized it has been given a name—apoptosis.

THE LIFE SPAN OF A CELL

Our body's cells contain chromosomes and telomeres within their nuclei that are essential for cell reproduction. Chromosomes contain the body's genetic information and influence our growth and development. Each time a cell reproduces, the chromosomes are copied identically into the new cell. Telomeres, however, are nongenetic material and appear to reproduce erratically with each cell division. There is evidence that the body's supply of telomeres is limited, and so our life span is genetically determined.

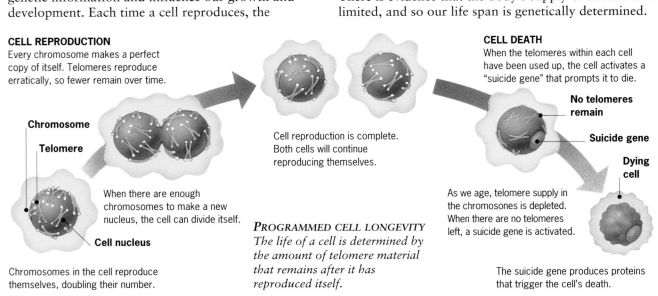

CELL REPRODUCTION
Every chromosome makes a perfect copy of itself. Telomeres reproduce erratically, so fewer remain over time.

Chromosome

Telomere

Cell nucleus

When there are enough chromosomes to make a new nucleus, the cell can divide itself.

Chromosomes in the cell reproduce themselves, doubling their number.

Cell reproduction is complete. Both cells will continue reproducing themselves.

PROGRAMMED CELL LONGEVITY
The life of a cell is determined by the amount of telomere material that remains after it has reproduced itself.

CELL DEATH
When the telomeres within each cell have been used up, the cell activates a "suicide gene" that prompts it to die.

No telomeres remain

Suicide gene

Dying cell

As we age, telomere supply in the chromosones is depleted. When there are no telomeres left, a suicide gene is activated.

The suicide gene produces proteins that trigger the cell's death.

The theory of accumulated damage is based on the notion that aging may be determined by an individual's lifestyle and environment. As a result of external damage, the immune system declines in strength, reducing the body's defenses against bacteria, viruses, and cancer. Other cell repair mechanisms also deteriorate, and a gradual buildup of toxins occurs. DNA, the blueprint of each cell, wears out over time, causing mistakes to occur in tissue and organ systems. This theory does not ignore preprogrammed cell death but argues that damage accumulation may affect the timing of it. In other words, by looking after ourselves we may delay some automatic aging processes. Most scientists believe that aging is a result of both preprogrammed cell death and accumulated damage to the cells.

PREPROGRAMMED AGING

The theory of preprogrammed aging revolves around cell behavior and hormone production; both of these essential functions in our body seem to operate according to fixed biological time frames.

Preprogrammed cell death

Scientists now know that the ability of cells to replicate and therefore sustain life is finite. Each DNA strand has a limited supply of telomeres, a nongenetic cellular material that is essential to the cell reproduction process. Every time a cell reproduces, we use up a little more of this material, until there are no telomeres left and cell reproduction ceases. Interestingly, cancer cells have found a way of replicating telomeres in order to continue their own reproduction. Scientists are currently investigating the possibility that cancer cells may provide a secret to postponing aging.

There are other aspects of cell aging. If any components of a cell are missing, it will become dysfunctional. Old cells have been shown to lack various genetic products. One of these is the Fos protein, made by the fos gene. The Fos protein alerts other genes to make the cell grow. Because aging cells lack this protein, other genes do not do their job, and the cell does not replicate.

There are many other genes that are equally critical to the life of a cell, such as the gene that produces the Apo-1 protein. This protein triggers the cell to die or undergo apoptosis when the time is right. There

are other similar "suicide" genes. Cells also have "rescue genes," such as the bcl-2 gene, which can postpone apoptosis. Some rescue genes are particularly important because they can inhibit the formation of free radicals, which have been identified as causal factors in diseases such as cancer. Free radicals are unstable oxygen molecules or atoms that form naturally in the body as a result of biochemical processes in cells. If too many free radicals build up, the body's natural antioxidants, or free radical fighters, cannot cope with them, and they can cause illness and disease.

It is the interaction between the different genes in your body's cells that determines their life span and therefore also determines the pace of your aging.

Hormones and aging

The fact that hormones decline naturally with age seems to indicate that aging and death are predetermined. The ones that most obviously decline are the sex hormones: testosterone in men and estrogen in women. A major reason for the reduced production of hormones is the declining efficiency of the hypothalamus. This is a gland in the brain that produces its own hormones and also controls the production of hormones elsewhere in the body. When the hypothalamus has been stimulated in laboratory animals, longevity has been increased by 50 percent.

Another hormone associated with aging is dehydroepiandrosterone (DHEA), which peaks at age 30 and declines to 10 percent of its peak by age 70. DHEA is a steroid that appears to control the action of the sex hormones. DHEA also blocks the negative

continued on page 22

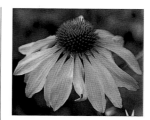

***ECHINACEA
(E. PURPUREA)***
Also known as purple coneflower, this North American herb is widely used for its ability to help ward off colds and flu and heal skin problems and yeast infections. It is also being studied for its possible effect on cancer cells and arthritis.

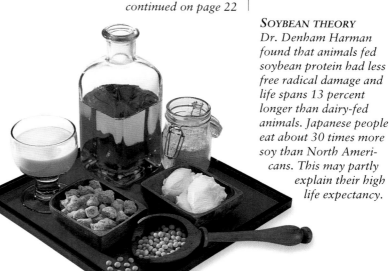

SOYBEAN THEORY
Dr. Denham Harman found that animals fed soybean protein had less free radical damage and life spans 13 percent longer than dairy-fed animals. Japanese people eat about 30 times more soy than North Americans. This may partly explain their high life expectancy.

The Geriatrician

The latter half of the 20th century saw a steady increase in life expectancy. Research into aging increased in tandem with this change and led to the development of a new branch of medicine devoted to the health and well-being of older people.

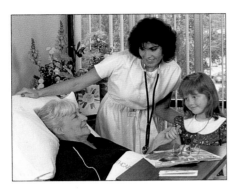

FAMILY HELP
Help from family members is often vital for older people to recuperate properly from illness or surgery. For this reason geriatricians often include family members in discussing aftercare.

EXPERT KNOWLEDGE
When an elderly patient is discharged from a hospital, a geriatrician makes sure that the patient fully understands his condition and any treatment that has been prescribed. This doctor may also give advice on what exercises or other self-care measures could be beneficial.

Gerontology is the scientific study of the aging process and old age itself, covering diverse sociological, biological, and medical issues. A geriatrician, or clinical gerontologist, is primarily concerned with the treatment and prevention of illness in older people but also manages their care in conjunction with their social needs. This includes helping others involved in the care of a patient—the spouse, a relative, or another caregiver. The principles of geriatric medicine are not based on a pathology of aging. Old age is not a disease that needs to be cured but a natural life process in which ill health is not inevitable.

What qualifications does a geriatrician have?
A geriatrician is a medical doctor who has undergone additional training in the specialty of gerontology. A physician working in the field will have extensive training in internal medicine and often in psychiatry as well.

How and why are people referred to a geriatrician?
A patient's first contact with a geriatrician may be by referral from a family doctor. This is usually in connection with specific conditions, such as Parkinson's disease and osteoporosis, which are common afflictions of older people. Alternatively, admission to a hospital—after a fall, for example—may mean automatic referral to a geriatrician if the patient is over a certain age.

Do you have to be in a hospital to be treated by a geriatrician?
Most major hospitals do have at least one geriatrician on staff, but hospitals are not the only places where they practice. Since patients are not admitted to a hospital unless their condition absolutely requires it, a geriatrician may be consulted long before a hospital stay is necessary.

People with ongoing but not critical conditions may be referred by a general practitioner to an outpatient clinic. Individuals suffering from more serious conditions or those who require round-the-clock care may benefit

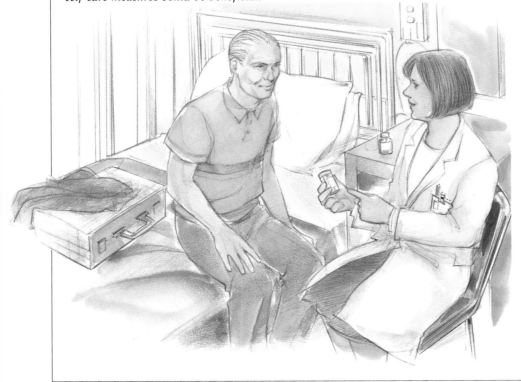

from attending a day care center. At the center a geriatrician is able to observe and monitor the day-to-day progress of patients to ensure they are receiving the best possible treatment. This also allows the individual to continue living at home, which for many people is an understandably emotional priority. Whenever possible, care is given in the manner that is least disruptive of the patient's life.

What is different about geriatric medicine?

Medical treatment of the elderly suffered in the past from the mistaken belief that old age inevitably leads to a reduction in quality of life and expectations of health—a belief often shared by the patients themselves. A geriatrician must establish with the patient the idea that when illness does occur, it can be treated.

A geriatrician sees a wide range of problems—physical, emotional, and neurological—and the divisions between categories are not always clearcut. Apparent mental deterioration or confusion may be caused by a physical problem—for example, loss of hearing or sight—rather than a reduction in mental faculty. Symptoms of illness in older adults do not present themselves as obviously as in younger people, which may pose difficulties for the geriatrician when making a diagnosis and determining treatment. For example, pain—the body's early warning system—is recognized less readily by older people. This often means that a disease may be further advanced by the time it is identified.

Older people are also more likely to have multiple problems, which can mask the causes of ill health, and drugs must be prescribed with great care to avoid dangerous interactions. It is essential to make sure that a secondary or underlying condition is not worsened by side effects caused by treatment of a more serious or obvious condition and that drugs do not create new problems.

Origins

Elie Metchnikoff (1845–1916) was one of the first scientists to study the cellular processes of aging. He coined the term *gerontology* in 1903 to describe his scientific study. A Russian bacteriologist, Metchnikoff joined the Pasteur Institute in Paris in 1888, where his work on immunology and cell research led to his sharing the Nobel Prize for medicine in 1908. His research into aging led to the rejection of the notion that old age was necessarily a time of ill health and dependence, and the discipline of geriatric medicine evolved.

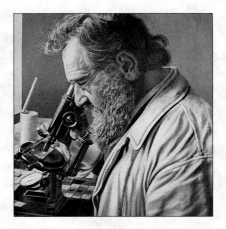

ELIE METCHNIKOFF
Metchnikoff was one of the first scientists to study the processes of aging and geriatric medicine.

WHAT YOU CAN DO AT HOME

One aim of a geriatrician is to help older people maintain their independence as long as possible. The active participation of the patient can make a real difference.

You can boost your health and chances of staying fitter longer by making sure you have regular medical examinations and are screened for common disorders (see pages 52–53). Consider having an influenza vaccination before the onset of winter. For future reference you should also keep a record of any drugs you are prescribed.

Making your home as safe as possible will help you remain independent. Adding safety rails and improving lighting may prove to be invaluable adaptations.

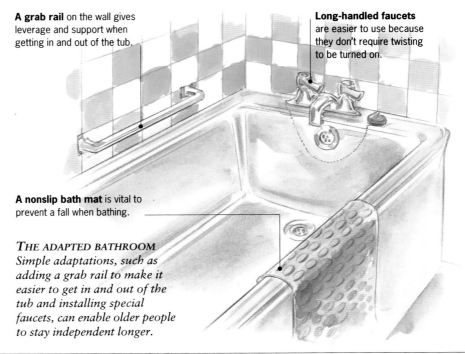

A grab rail on the wall gives leverage and support when getting in and out of the tub.

Long-handled faucets are easier to use because they don't require twisting to be turned on.

A nonslip bath mat is vital to prevent a fall when bathing.

THE ADAPTED BATHROOM
Simple adaptations, such as adding a grab rail to make it easier to get in and out of the tub and installing special faucets, can enable older people to stay independent longer.

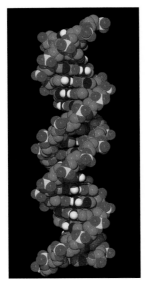

THE KEY TO LIFE
DNA contains the genetic information that determines how each cell develops and functions. Little was known about a link between DNA and old age until the 1970s, when Russian theorist Alexei Olovnikov set out to prove his theory that the shortening of DNA strands was the key to aging and cell death.

effects of some of the hormones produced when a person is under stress. Ongoing research has indicated that administering DHEA may slow down aging and also increase longevity, but the findings are as yet inconclusive.

Research has also been done on the effect that growth hormone has on aging. This hormone stimulates the thymus gland, which is essential for the function of the immune system and helps to build bones, heal wounds, and maintain the health of muscles and organs. Experiments carried out by Joseph Meites in 1990, published in the *Review of Biological Research in Aging*, showed that when growth hormone was given to people 60 to 70 years old, aging was not only stopped but actually reversed in some biological functions. Further investigation is still required, however, because dangerous side effects were observed. Nevertheless, it is clear that the continued health of the immune system is essential to reducing the effects of aging. A healthy diet and regular exercise will ensure a healthy immune system that will fight disease and attacks from free radicals.

Melatonin, a hormone that regulates biorhythms, has in recent years been linked with slowing aging. Although melatonin has been used to extend longevity in rats, the results are not conclusive, and there is no evidence that it would work for humans. There are no regulations governing melatonin production, so it is inadvisable to take it without consulting your doctor first.

ACCUMULATED DAMAGE THEORY

As cells grow older and experience normal wear and tear, they accumulate damage. Human cells can deal with a certain amount of harm, but over time they lose the ability to effectively repair themselves. Some of this damage is caused by environmental and lifestyle factors that cause free radical buildup. There are several cell components, or molecules, involved in the aging process that may be affected by damage accumulation, including proteins, sugars, and DNA. Cumulative damage processes increase with age because of damage to genes, but why this happens is not known.

Heat shock genes

When tissues undergo extreme stress, such as a burn, so-called heat-shock genes produce proteins to repair the cells. Different types of heat-shock genes respond to different stresses. For instance, one type will respond to psychological stress, whereas another type will respond to ingestion of poisons. There is yet another heat-shock gene that responds to free radicals.

As we grow older, this heat-shock response becomes impaired because fewer proteins are produced by the genes and those that remain become less effective. This may explain why older people are less able to withstand acute environmental stresses. The disrepair that builds up causes aging. Avoiding or controlling all forms of stress may therefore be very important in relieving this buildup.

ENVIRONMENTAL ATTACK

The body produces free radicals, scavengers that damage cells, as natural by-products of metabolism—chemical changes that take place in cells to create energy for the body's functions. However, external factors in the modern world also contribute to the production of free radicals. Hydrocarbons and nitrogen oxides in the air, caused by pollution such as car exhaust fumes; increased radiation from the sun, caused by thinning of the ozone layer; cigarette smoke; and industrial chemicals—all increase the production of free radicals.

OZONE DEPLETION
The dark blue area in this picture denotes a vast hole in the ozone layer over Antarctica that lets harmful radiation reach the earth.

DAMAGE CAUSED BY FREE RADICALS

A free radical is formed when certain molecules within cells encounter oxygen and break apart. The fragments, or free radicals, are unstable and bind with the nearest molecule. This damages the genetic code within that cell, causing it to become deformed or even to die. Antioxidants protect cells by binding harmlessly with free radicals once they are produced, rendering them impotent.

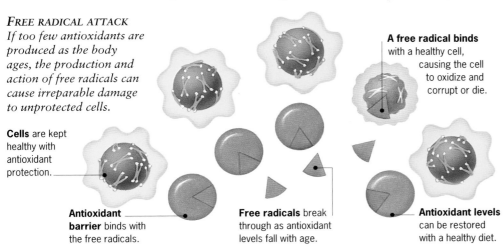

FREE RADICAL ATTACK
If too few antioxidants are produced as the body ages, the production and action of free radicals can cause irreparable damage to unprotected cells.

A free radical binds with a healthy cell, causing the cell to oxidize and corrupt or die.

Cells are kept healthy with antioxidant protection.

Antioxidant barrier binds with the free radicals.

Free radicals break through as antioxidant levels fall with age.

Antioxidant levels can be restored with a healthy diet.

Free radicals and aging

Free radicals are also considered crucial in aging. They lead to the damage or death of cells because they corrupt the mitochondria DNA (mitochondria are the cells' energy source). As people grow older, the damage done by free radicals becomes more widespread. Free radicals also damage proteins and fats, causing such problems as atherosclerosis (see page 55) or cancer (see pages 74–76). What researchers want to know is why free radicals build up. It is thought that the body's natural antioxidants (vitamins A, C, and E, as well as some minerals and flavonoids) decrease because the genes that produce them switch off or become damaged with age. There is now a great deal of evidence that the damage caused by free radicals can be limited or prevented by eating foods rich in antioxidants (see page 86).

Glucose cross-linking

Many molecules in the body need glucose added to them to function, a process known as glucose cross-linking or glycosylation. There are various proteins that supervise this process. If the molecules do not attach to glucose or if the glucose attaches to the wrong molecules, the body will not be able to function properly. For reasons not fully understood, this process begins to go wrong as we get older. Glucose attaches to the wrong molecules, such as proteins or DNA, creating complex and unnecessary structures in cells called advanced glycosylation end products. It is thought that the accumulation of these products in cells is associated with such diseases as diabetes. The cell mechanisms that would usually fight these end products seem to deteriorate with age, supporting the idea that aging is associated with genetic breakdown. Scientists are now investigating how factors such as diet may be implicated in this problem.

CAN SCIENCE REVERSE AGING?

While research into the genetics of aging continues to throw light on the processes involved, it is already very clear the extent to which we can prevent much of the damage to cells traditionally seen as an inevitable part of growing older. Reducing exposure to free radicals by stopping smoking, for example, is a simple but very effective antiaging strategy. Similarly, paying attention to diet, especially consuming more fruits and vegetables, can bring real dividends. Even though science may yet unlock the cellular "fountain of youth," we already hold in our own hands the power to make our old age healthier and more active, comfortable, and fulfilling.

RESCUE GENE
Bcl–2 is one of the genes that scientists are investigating to better understand aging, because it prevents apoptosis, or cell death.

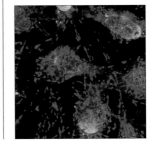

FACTORS THAT AFFECT AGING

Many biological factors can influence the pace of aging, but much research is being focused today on general lifestyle issues, such as diet, exercise, and mental attitude.

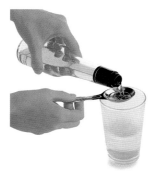

VERMONT FOLK REMEDY
Dr. D.C. Jarvis, the author of a book called Folk Medicine, *noted in 1858 the longevity of Vermont apple farmers, who worked well into their seventies and eighties. The farmers put this down to taking 2 tablespoons of cider vinegar and honey in a cup of hot water every morning. The remedy keeps the body slightly acidic, which they believed helped to ward off a range of conditions, including high blood pressure, arthritis, hay fever, and weight gain.*

The environment we live in and the way we take care of ourselves have an influence on the way we age. Our genetic inheritance also plays an important role, but scientists are looking increasingly at the larger picture and recognizing the interaction between genes and lifestyle. For example, many researchers are interested in the fact that women, in general, live longer than men. Life expectancy in the United States is about 79 years for women, 72 years for men. In Canada the figures are 82 years for women, 75 years for men. There are many theories to explain this gender gap,

none of them proven. Some gerontologists believe that female longevity is associated with women having two X chromosomes (men have one X and one Y chromosome). Others speculate that female sex hormones may extend longevity or that male sex hormones may decrease it, but there is no conclusive evidence for any of these theories.

Ultimately, however, lifestyle issues seem to be of greatest significance in the gender difference. Women are less likely to work in environmentally dangerous professions and are more open to alternative therapies and lifestyle improvements. Men are statistically

---

A HEALTHIER ENVIRONMENT

Improvements in the environment since the early 19th century have significantly bettered the health of city dwellers in North America. These include better

water, sewer, and sanitation facilities, clean-air laws, and some clearance of slums. However, industrial and traffic pollution still poses risks.

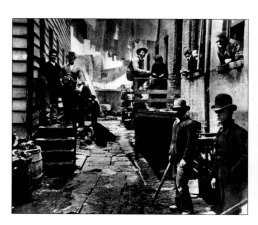

EARLY 19TH CENTURY
Millions of people lived in cramped, dirty conditions with poor sanitation. Epidemics such as cholera and typhoid were common.

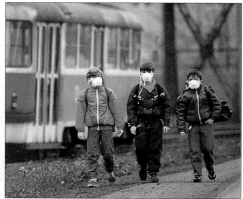

TODAY
Air pollution caused by emissions from factories and vehicle traffic continue to threaten public health in cities.

more likely to sustain serious injuries or encounter acts of violence; they are far more likely to die from car accidents, homicide, and suicide, for example. Men are also more susceptible to illnesses that may have a lifestyle component to them, such as heart attack, stroke, and cancer.

Our genetic inheritance will, to a degree, determine our susceptibility to many of the diseases associated with aging. For instance, high cholesterol levels and high blood pressure (factors in heart disease and stroke), as well as Alzheimer's disease and some cancers, have a genetic component. However, research has increasingly revealed the extent to which healthy living might prevent some of these conditions.

Lifestyle also seems to be more important than racial background. Although from time to time reports of people living to 120 years or more in far-flung corners of the earth come to light, these stories have not been substantiated because of incomplete or nonexistent birth records. There is no scientific evidence to suggest that any race is more susceptible to aging than any other. Such lifestyle factors as diet and exercise are far more relevant. For example, the diets in Japan, China, and Mediterranean countries are lower in fat than the typical North American diet, and fewer people in these countries die of heart disease. People who have remained active throughout their lives and include exercise in their daily routines also tend to live longer. So exactly what are the factors that influence aging?

MENTAL ATTITUDES

State of mind and vulnerability to stress can have a profound effect on an individual's well-being. A new branch of research called psychoneuroimmunology (PNI) has shown that mental state directly affects the immune system. Scientists Robert Ader and Nicholas Cohen gave rats saccharin-flavored water containing a drug to suppress immune system functioning. When the sweetened water was later given to the rats without the drug, their immune systems were still affected.

Researchers Ron Glaser and Janice Kiecolt-Glaser demonstrated in 1993 that stress has a direct influence on the immune system of humans when they identified a connection between a nerve and a lymphocyte (a white blood cell). It is believed that thought patterns and moods can trigger the

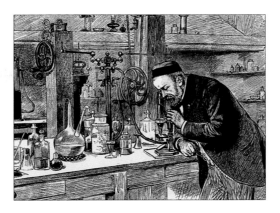

release of hormones that then have a wide-ranging effect on vital body systems. The researchers produced evidence showing that even some minor stresses, such as arguing with a spouse or trying to complete a frustrating task, can cause enough stress to have a detrimental effect on health. Learning to cope positively with stress may therefore help slow the aging process.

LIFESTYLE

Scientists believe that increased longevity will more likely be achieved through better living conditions than improvements in medical treatment. In 1900 only 4 percent of the North American population was 65 or over. Better housing, health care, and sanitation and more awareness of preventive medicine increased that figure to 12.5 percent in 1996. During the 20th century, average life expectancy increased by nearly 30 years, in part due to a lowering of the infant mortality rate.

There is still much room for improvement, however, because pollution, sedentary lifestyles, and high-fat diets continue to pose risks to health. Illnesses associated with aging, such as heart disease and cancer, escalated in the latter half of the 20th century. It is now known that specific factors, like regular, balanced meals, weight control, adequate sleep, regular exercise, and abstinence from smoking all help to slow aging and prevent disease. Not surprisingly, drinking alcohol to excess and abusing drugs accelerate aging and can shorten the length of our lives considerably.

Socioeconomic status is also a major factor in aging. People with a higher standard of living and better health care live longer. Occupation seems to have an influence as well. Research suggests that, after dangerous occupations are factored out, the occupations with higher life expectancies seem

LOUIS PASTEUR
French chemist Louis Pasteur was the first to prove a link between microorganisms and the processes of decay and fermentation. His research into vaccination and pasteurization—the sterilization process named after him—led to major advances in control of diseases.

OCCUPATION AND AGE
In 1974 a survey carried out by the Metropolitan Life Insurance Company found that conductors are likely to live the longest. Their death rate was 38 percent lower than the average for the general population.

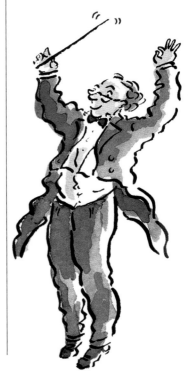

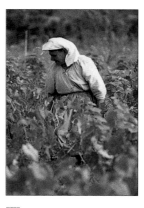

WORKING FOR THE FAMILY
Many agricultural workers in essentially agrarian communities work well past the accepted Western retirement age because of the familial and social requirements imposed by living off the land.

to be those that are personally fulfilling, which could range from making pottery to being a corporate executive. Those who experience a great deal of stress at work, with little control over their workload, suffer more stress-related illness and, it is thought, accelerated aging. It may be that a sense of purpose and self-worth are as important in longevity as physical health; cultural factors could also be very important.

CULTURAL PERCEPTIONS OF AGE
It has been a common assumption in the West that aging involves a gradual withdrawal from the world into passivity, dependence, and decreasing usefulness in society. In fact, most older people continue to lead lives filled with challenges, but they have to respond to social and physical changes with imagination and determination.

Some other cultures have not had such a passive view of growing older. The ancient Romans revered the wisdom and experience that age brought. The name of their governing body, the senatus, was derived from the Latin *senex*, which means "old."

Today the Chakma people of Bangladesh live in three-generation family units. The grandparents play active roles in bringing up the children, and respect for elders is paramount in society. This family structure, common in many Buddhist and Hindu societies, is found all over Asia and India. The Native American Choctaw tribe is also led by the oldest members, who are beloved and greatly respected. This pattern is repeated across many traditional Native American societies. In Japan, "Respect for the Aged Day" is celebrated as a national holiday every September.

SIGNS OF AGING
When a wrinkle appears on a Chinese woman's face, it is greeted with celebration by her daughters and granddaughters. Wrinkles are seen as a sign of wisdom and growing status.

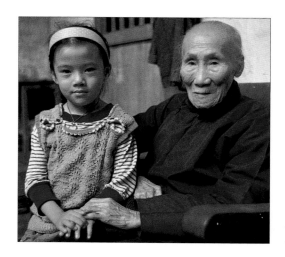

Pathway to health
Making sure that you stay young at heart is an excellent way of coping with the challenges of growing older. You should remain in control of your life as much as possible. As long as you are capable of making decisions, continue to do so rather than allow well-meaning friends or relatives to make them for you.

Stay in touch with other people. Social isolation is known to increase the risk of illness and death. Daily contact with friends can do wonders for your emotional health and general sense of well-being. This is especially important if you have recently suffered a bereavement.

It is never too late to learn. Every few months, resolve to achieve something new. Goals might include learning a new skill or trying a new exercise. The sense of achievement will build your confidence and keep you feeling young.

There are some indications that cultural perceptions have an effect on memory retention during the aging process, although some memory function does appear to decline with age no matter what. Tests carried out by two psychologists, Becca Levy and Ellen Langer, and published in 1994 demonstrated that elderly Chinese people performed as well as younger Chinese when given a memory test. The elderly Chinese did not expect to decline significantly in mental ability or social status as they grew older, whereas older American participants tested in the same way were outstripped by their younger counterparts. The findings led Levy and Langer to conclude that cultural beliefs about aging might serve as a self-fulfilling prophecy. If the older Americans had had positive expectations about aging similar to those of their Chinese contemporaries, their memory function might have shown a much less marked deterioration.

Increasingly, Westerners are beginning to challenge traditional stereotypes that exist about aging and to understand that their health and well-being, and therefore their rate of aging, may be harmed by a negative attitude toward life.

DEALING WITH THE CHANGES OF AGING

Dealing positively with the physical and emotional changes that occur as part of the aging process can bring you immense benefits in terms of your lifestyle and general well-being.

Many people have a negative view of aging because they are focusing on the physical changes that are associated with growing older—wrinkles and stiff joints, for instance. But aging also involves the accumulation of knowledge and experience, which can be of real value in relationships and in helping yourself and others make satisfying life choices.

PHYSICAL CHANGE

In addition to changes in appearance, other less obvious physical changes take place with advancing years. Many of these physical indicators of biological age have been labeled biomarkers. But several biomarkers are not necessarily linked to chronological age (see chart on page 28), and a number of them can be positively altered by diet and exercise.

As we grow older, there is a gradual decline in the function of all body tissues, including bones, muscles, and internal organs like the heart, liver, intestines, lungs, kidneys, and brain. However, regular exercise can dramatically improve the functioning of muscles and other tissues.

The ratio of muscle to fat alters in favor of fat as we age, which may be linked to a reduction in the body's basal metabolic rate (BMR). Your BMR is the amount of energy your body uses to fuel its functions. These changes can lead to increased weight and weight-related illness. Exercise can help by improving the ratio of muscle to fat, which in turn improves the BMR because muscle burns more energy than fat. It may also be necessary to pay more attention to diet to help control weight.

By middle age there are declines in hearing, vision, and response times to mental and physical challenges. However, there is evidence that avoiding environmental damage can reduce age-related problems with the senses. (Chapter 3 provides more detail on age-related illnesses and how to avoid them and minimize their effects.)

Although the latter part of life is associated with a reduction in physical capacity, this is less dramatic than many believe. The technology of developed countries has made physical labor much less important, so there is no longer any need to equate old age with an inability to work and contribute to society. Experience gained over the years gives older people a clear advantage in many situations over those younger than they are. Often it is only negative cultural factors that prevent older people from achieving their full potential. Breaking down such barriers will allow you to realize just how much you can influence your chances of enjoying a strong mind and body in later years. With a

Accepting changes
Some changes are inevitable as you age. Graying hair, poorer eyesight and hearing, and menopause in women can't be prevented. But there are things you can do to minimize other physical changes. Limiting your exposure to sun will delay the appearance of wrinkles; keeping fit will help counteract a decrease in sexual desire; and continuing curiosity and enthusiasm for life will keep your mind active.

A NEW LEASE ON LIFE

Following her roles in the television series *The Avengers* and the James Bond film *Goldfinger*, Honor Blackman was seen to represent the independent woman of the 1960s.

After years of relative obscurity, her career was given a new lease on life when television roles reaffirmed her fame as a timeless beauty. Honor Blackman showed that attractiveness is not exclusively associated with youth and that a woman can age naturally and gracefully without losing her appeal.

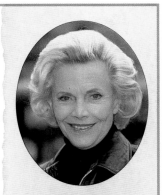

HONOR BLACKMAN
Enduring sex appeal helped Honor Blackman maintain a successful acting career.

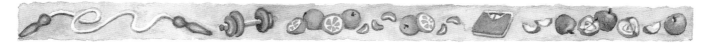

BIOMARKERS

Aging is an intractable fact of life that affects all our body's functions. Can the process be slowed or reversed? The answer is yes, according to researchers William Evans and Irwin Rosenberg at Tufts University.

They identified 10 biomarkers—critical factors that influence physical vitality, which the individual can alter through diet and a regular program of aerobics and flexibility and strength training.

BIOMARKER	WHAT THE EFFECTS OF AGING ARE	WHAT YOU CAN DO
Muscle mass	Lean body mass typically declines.	Exercise to maintain muscle mass; this will also increase aerobic capacity and strength.
Strength	There is gradual loss of muscle strength, leading to a reduction in mobility and general fitness, as well as a loss of bone density.	Training with weights or some other form of resistance will increase your strength.
Basal metabolic rate (BMR)	BMR usually slows down with age, causing an increase in weight .	Increase your muscle mass. This will raise your BMR and help to prevent gaining of excess weight.
Body fat percentage (fat to muscle ratio)	A higher fat to muscle ratio increases the risk of heart disease and stroke.	Increase your BMR and muscle mass by keeping active to reduce any health risks.
Aerobic capacity	A sedentary lifestyle decreases the efficiency of the heart and lungs.	Do exercise like jogging, brisk walking, aerobic dance, or cycling to help your heart use oxygen more efficiently.
Blood pressure	Blood pressure may rise with age. High blood pressure increases the risk of stroke and heart disease.	Even moderate forms of regular exercise, such as walking, can help control blood pressure.
Blood sugar tolerance	Your body may become less efficient in controlling blood sugar as you age. This increases the risk of developing Type II diabetes.	Maintaining a diet rich in high-fiber complex carbohydrates, such as whole-grain bread and cereal, will help keep your blood sugar levels steady.
Cholesterol	An unhealthy diet and sedentary lifestyle can increase levels of "bad" LDL cholesterol and decrease the "good" HDL cholesterol necessary for hormone production.	Cholesterol levels can be controlled by reducing saturated fats and increasing soluble fiber in the diet and exercising regularly.
Bone density	There is a decline in the mineral content of bones.	Doing weight-bearing exercise and eating foods rich in calcium will help maintain bone density.
Body temperature regulation	There is a decline in the effectiveness of the body's temperature-regulating mechanism..	Regular exercise can help the body react better to changes in temperature.

positive attitude and knowledge of your body's needs, you can maintain good health well into your later years.

SOCIAL CHANGE

As you grow older, your role in society will undergo many changes. After your children grow up, you will have less involvement with their activities and more time for other interests. After retirement you will have to find new ways of occupying your time, by joining organizations or participating in volunteer work, for example. Some people also find they have a renewed interest in religion at this time of life.

Eventually you will be referred to as a retiree and a senior citizen; these labels carry both positive and negative implications. Such changes require flexibility and a positive attitude on your part to accommodate them in your life.

If you become a grandparent, you may find yourself once again involved in raising children. Many people enjoy this role immensely, whereas others feel it is an infringement on their freedom. You may also wonder if the younger generations come from the same planet as you do if you cannot understand their ways or are having difficulty communicating with them.

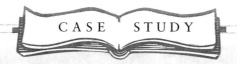
An Older Widower

Following the loss of a spouse, loneliness and grief are often accompanied by more incidences of illness, as well as an increase in the physical and emotional changes associated with aging. Being able to overcome grief in a constructive way is important to resuming a full life and protecting yourself against ill health.

Evan, aged 69, lost his wife, Cynthia, to cancer three months ago. They had been married for 40 years, and he feels completely grief stricken. Since she died, he has been unable to sleep properly and has no appetite and no motivation to prepare food for himself. Cynthia did most of the shopping and cooking, and Evan feels unable to organize things himself. He does not eat regularly, and although his children invite him for meals, he eats very little. For most of his life Evan has been healthy and active but now feels lethargic and unwell. He has been having palpitations, chest pains, and stomach pains. And he has no interest in socializing or going bowling with his friends as he once did.

WHAT SHOULD EVAN DO?

Evan's physical symptoms, as well as his poor diet and lack of activity, are most likely a result of his grief. However, to make sure he has no serious medical problems, he should see his doctor for a checkup. He then needs to find constructive ways to deal with his grief, even though he has little motivation to do so. Seeing a grief counselor may help. Evan could also discuss his feelings with a close friend. He should ask a friend or one of his children to help him shop and cook until he gets back on his feet. He should also get out of the house as often as possible, perhaps by doing volunteer work, and resume a normal daily routine. Keeping busy is one of the best ways to cope with grief and depression.

Action Plan

DIET
Make an effort to eat properly and regularly, even if appetite is lacking; otherwise, long-term health could be put in danger.

EXERCISE
Go for a walk every day to break out of lethargy and increase energy levels. Resume the weekly bowling game.

EMOTIONAL HEALTH
Seek support and companionship from close friends and perhaps meet with a grief counselor. Try to socialize more to break the cycle of depression and grief.

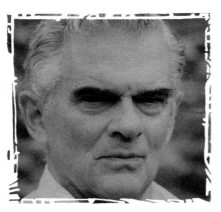

EMOTIONAL HEALTH
The emotions that follow the death of a loved one can cause many physical symptoms.

DIET
Depression often suppresses appetite, as well as the motivation to prepare food. The results of an inadequate diet can compound health problems.

EXERCISE
Sadness and grief can make one lethargic and uninterested in any kind of activity. Exercise, however, is a very effective way to feel better emotionally.

HOW THINGS TURNED OUT FOR EVAN

Lucy, a longtime friend of Evan and Cynthia, realized that Evan was not coping. She persuaded him to see a doctor, who confirmed that he had no major medical problems but needed to exercise and eat better. Lucy took Evan shopping and showed him how to make a few easy meals. Her visits also gave him an opportunity to talk about his loss, which helped ease his grief. After a few months Evan felt he was on the road to recovery.

FIGHTING STRESS
Being able to take care of themselves is an important factor in reducing stress for many older people. Self-defense classes enhance self-confidence and independence by showing how to defend oneself through good technique rather than strength, and they help maintain fitness at the same time.

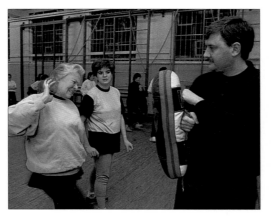

AGING AND STRESS

Stress is a fact of life. Excessive amounts of stress can make people age more quickly or become ill, but not if the mechanisms they use to deal with their problems are effective. Hans Selye, researching the effects of stress during the 1930s, declared that stress-related illnesses were caused by faulty adaptation reactions. People who have poor coping skills tend to suffer from depression and anxiety and are physically ill more often. Those who feel they can deal with whatever comes their way are often happier and physically much healthier.

CHECKLIST
It has been proven that the body's immune system is affected by our levels of stress, so learning effective coping mechanisms is important.

✔ *Eliminate any negative thoughts that adversely affect your mood and focus on positive emotions.*

✔ *Identify any sources of stress and consciously limit the effects they have on your day-to-day life.*

✔ *Learn to relax, either through relaxation techniques or hobbies, in order to deal effectively with stressful situations.*

✔ *Do not turn to such unhealthy crutches as cigarettes, alcohol, and overeating to deal with stress; these create their own problems.*

✔ *Learn to resolve your difficulties by nonaggressively airing your emotions and problems.*

Physical ailments that can be brought on or exacerbated by stress are common among the elderly. These include arthritis, fibrositis, neckache, backache, high blood pressure, and irritable bowel syndrome. Learning to recognize and acknowledge negative emotions is the first step to having greater control over these and other stress-related problems. If you are aware of the stress caused by certain situations, you will be more likely to notice the effect they have on your physical health. Be honest if you are unhappy with a situation. Repressing your emotions will not make them go away; they will simply manifest themselves in other ways, such as physical aches and pains.

Taking up an activity that allows a vent for these feelings is a more effective way to cope than passively tolerating stressful situations. This can be anything from a sport or outdoor pursuit that you enjoy to a creative outlet, such as painting or music. Meditation classes can also help you learn how to relax and how to identify times when you are feeling stressed. You will find that developing more effective coping mechanisms for the stresses you are bound to encounter occasionally can also provide considerable pain relief for many physical conditions.

A loss of confidence and self-esteem commonly afflicts people in middle age. Signs of aging become more noticeable and are often accompanied by major life changes, like children leaving home, menopause, and the death of friends or a partner. Questions such as "Am I still sexually desirable?" "What have I achieved in life so far?" and "What does the future hold for me?" can give rise to concern and stress and thus adversely affect physical health, causing a downward spiral of negativity that can be difficult to break. Doing something positive for your health is vital for your physical and emotional well-being; feeling physically better will boost your self-esteem and improve your mental outlook.

It is important to remember that failing health and illness are not inevitable consequences of aging. It is true that the body will become physically older and that your appearance will change, but this need not affect your abilities or mental capacity. A positive mental attitude and a high level of self-esteem, coupled with living an active and satisfying life, will be reflected by continuing health and happiness in later life.

CHAPTER 2

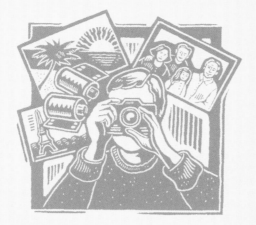

A POSITIVE OUTLOOK

Aging brings with it changes in family routines, friendships, and often work and finances—not all of which are necessarily welcome. If you remain active and maintain a high level of self-esteem, good relationships with family and friends, and a positive attitude toward life, you can help yourself grow into a healthy and happy old age.

CHANGING LIFESTYLES

Teenagers have to undergo life changes without fully expecting or understanding them, but older people can use their experience and wisdom to anticipate change and prepare for it.

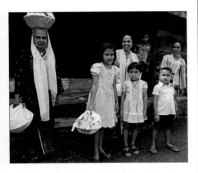

EXTENDED FAMILY
In many cultures extended families provide support for both younger and older members. In societies in which this is not the case, people are starting to recognize the benefits of shared responsibility for child care and finances across the generations.

NEVER TOO OLD
or too young to learn. Teaching a skill to a younger person can be rewarding and a valuable learning experience for both of you.

For most people advancing age brings not only physical changes but also changes in work, finances, lifestyle, and social relationships. Their effects on you will depend to a great extent on your personal circumstances, but it is vital to prepare for them as much as possible. For example, your income will probably drop when you retire. If you push this fact to the back of your mind—perhaps because you don't want to think about retirement until it happens—you may realize too late that you should have done more to prepare for the future while you were working.

ANTICIPATING LIFE CHANGES

Change of any kind can be difficult to cope with, but you will find it much easier to adjust if you have readied yourself psychologically and have taken whatever practical steps you can. If you allow change to creep up on you unnoticed or worry about your circumstances without confronting them, there is a good chance you will cope badly. Think ahead; identify the probable changes in your life over the coming months and years and plan how you are going to deal with them. If you adopt an optimistic outlook, you will be able to work out ways to minimize any drawbacks and maximize any advantages that these changes may bring.

GIVING UP WORK

As your retirement date approaches, you will probably have mixed emotions about leaving your job. You may be looking forward to the prospect of quitting work and enjoying your freedom, but this may be tinged with sadness, a sense of loss, and perhaps nervousness about what the future holds. You might not want to retire at all, in which case leaving your job will be difficult and stressful unless you resolve to put the past behind you and make a new start.

If you have worries about retiring, don't be afraid to admit them. Discuss them with your partner, your colleagues, or friends. Friends who have themselves retired can give you invaluable advice based on their own personal experiences.

Whatever your feelings may be about retirement, there are a number of ways in which you can ease the transition from working to not working. As your retirement date nears—whether it's a long-planned-for event or comes suddenly through ill health or redundancy—try to prepare yourself emotionally for your new way of life. Get used to the idea of being a retired person, of being in control of your life in a way that you could never be when you were working.

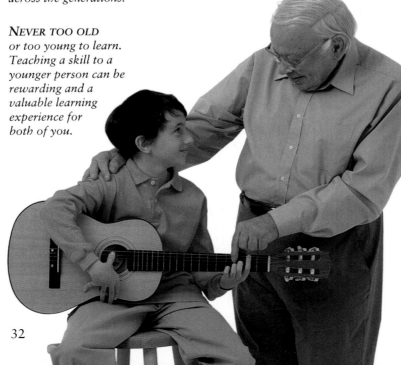

ADJUSTING TO RETIREMENT

If your job has been the center of your life for many years, retirement can be very stressful. In order to lessen the shock of leaving your job, take time to think about what you enjoy about your work and plan retirement activities that meet these needs. For example, if you enjoy teamwork and cooperating with people to achieve a goal, you might consider joining a volunteer group. If you like planning and organizing, perhaps you could play a more prominent role in clubs and societies. If you enjoy instructing and advising people, think about tutoring or teaching a course at a community college. These projects are a good way to remain actively involved with your community and pass on your skills to younger people.

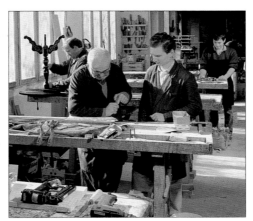

THE VALUE OF EXPERIENCE
Many older people volunteer to participate in training workshops, passing on their knowledge to younger generations to show them how to deal with work or social problems.

If your sense of self-identity has been closely associated with your work, remember that leaving your job is a change of occupation, not a change of personality.

If you would prefer to make a gradual exit from your working life, ask if your employer would be willing to let you work part-time during the last few months or weeks before you retire. Or, you might be able to work part-time after you have retired, filling in for colleagues who are sick or on leave. Before taking up any of these options, check that your pension rights will not be affected.

PLANNING YOUR RETIREMENT
If you simply drift into retirement, you risk letting it be something over which you have little or no control. This option might work out well if you are someone whose needs are few and who is happy doing nothing. But if you are not, you run the risk of an unfulfilling and even unhappy retirement, perhaps dogged by boredom and money problems.

A planned retirement can be an active and rewarding experience. Planning for it—in full consultation with your partner if you have one—gives you the opportunity to organize your finances and work out how you are going to spend your time. It also puts you more in control of your future, which in turn will boost your self-confidence and make retirement something to look forward to with pleasure rather than anxiety.

If you feel you need help with retirement planning, consider taking a preretirement course. These courses are designed to guide you through the emotional, financial, and practical aspects of retirement. They are given by some volunteer organizations, insurance firms, and pension management companies. Many large companies also provide them for their retiring employees.

PLANNING FOR FINANCIAL CHANGE
Ideally, you should plan for retirement by investing in a savings plan that will provide you with income to supplement your company pension and Social Security or Old Age Security. Whether or not you have this additional income to look forward to, there are a number of steps you can take before retiring to balance income and spending.

Clear as many debts as possible so you will not be burdened with large repayments on loans or credit cards. If you have a mortgage, pay it off if you can. If you plan to stay in your present home, have any major renovations—such as rewiring or a new roof—done and paid for while you are still working.

Before you can make realistic plans for your retirement, you must have a clear picture of what your financial position is likely to be. You must know what kind of pension you have; an index-linked pension will keep pace with the rate of inflation, whereas the value of a fixed-income pension will erode

Aging population
Thanks to higher standards of living and better health care, people are living longer today, and older people now make up a significant part of the population in most developed countries. In the United States, for example, the percentage of people over 65 has tripled since 1900, from just over 4 percent to nearly 13 percent. The country with the highest proportion of older people is Sweden, where more than 17 percent of the population is over 65.

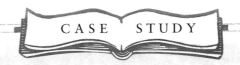
A Redundant Accountant

People who are laid off late in their working lives usually expect that they will soon find other work, but their hopes are often dashed. Their inability to find a job is usually no reflection on their abilities but on the reluctance of many companies to hire older workers. Nonetheless, older job seekers can quickly become demoralized and lose their sense of self-worth.

Dawn, 53, worked in the accounting department of a medium-sized company for over 30 years. A year ago the company was taken over, and her department was relocated to another town. Dawn took voluntary redundancy because she did not want to move, even though two of her colleagues who were also close friends decided to relocate. She expected to find another job quite easily because of her excellent qualifications and experience, but one application after another was turned down without an explanation—she suspects because of her age. She is financially secure, thanks to her severance settlement and savings, but feels rejected and is becoming increasingly isolated and depressed.

WHAT SHOULD DAWN DO?

Dawn should accept the fact that her expectations of getting another full-time job on her previous level are perhaps unrealistic and look for part-time or volunteer work instead. If she adopts a positive approach, she will see that working part-time has some advantages; it will make her feel useful again, restore her faith in herself, and leave her with enough energy and time to take up new interests.

She needs to rebuild her social life, which dwindled when two of her best friends moved away. She might make new friends through part-time work, but she should also consider widening her circle by joining a club that reflects her interests and/or attending evening classes.

Action Plan

LIFESTYLE
Take up activities that will help her to make new friends. Possibly join a club or enroll in some evening classes.

WORK
Be more realistic about employment prospects. Look for a part-time job or get involved with volunteer work.

EMOTIONAL HEALTH
Restore self-confidence by accepting that being turned down for a job does not diminish her value or potential.

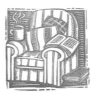

LIFESTYLE
Lack of an active social life can increase the feelings of isolation that are often brought on by unemployment.

WORK
It is easy to overestimate the chances of finding a similar job after accepting voluntary redundancy.

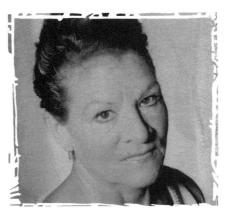

EMOTIONAL HEALTH
Being unemployed can undermine self-confidence, which may lead to anxiety and depression.

HOW THINGS TURNED OUT FOR DAWN

Dawn found a part-time job doing the accounting for a local company two days a week and is looking for similar work to do on one or two other days. She has taken up pottery in an evening class and is pleasantly surprised by her skill. She has also made friends with a couple of fellow students. Having survived a very difficult period, she feels increasingly confident and optimistic about this new phase in her life.

gradually. If you have changed jobs, you may also have pensions from different sources that you must claim, such as funds that remain frozen in a former employer's or a personal pension plan.

Widows and widowers are usually entitled to all or some of their spouse's pension, although divorced people may or may not have a similar entitlement. You should check the company's policy.

One important decision you will have to make is when to start claiming your government pension. In Canada the universal Old Age Security and the earnings-related Canada and Quebec pension Plans (CPP/QPP) are payable at age 65. Your CPP/QPP benefits can begin at age 60, but payments will be 70 percent of what you would receive at age 65. If you put off collecting until you are 70 years old, your payments will be 130 percent of what you would have received at age 65. The situation is similar in the United States; you can begin claiming Social Security benefits at age 62, but the earlier you begin payments, the lower they will be.

Find out if you qualify for any government benefits other than a pension. In Canada Old Age Security pensioners with little or no other income may qualify for a Guaranteed Income Supplement. In many U.S. communities senior citizens pay lower property taxes if their income is at a certain level. Utility companies in many American regions also grant special rates to retirees. Add to this figure other expected earnings, such as income from savings or investments.

A NEW LEASE ON LIFE

Born in 1912, Englishwoman Mary Wesley held several diverse jobs in her younger years, including one in the War Office during the Second World War. After her husband's death Mary took up writing in an effort to avoid financial difficulties. She published her first novel, *Jumping the Queue*, at the age of 70 and continued to write and publish several more, including *The Camomile Lawn*, which was adapted for television in 1991.

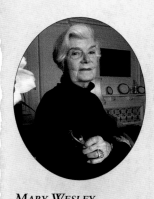

MARY WESLEY
Although Wesley became a novelist late in life, her work has received much recognition.

If you plan to work after your retirement, be cautious about including your pay in long-term income calculations because you cannot be sure how long you will continue working. Remember too that your pension is regarded as taxable income and take this into account.

Next, calculate your probable expenditures, taking account of how your spending will change when you stop working. Once you know what your essential expenditures will be, you can look for ways to economize if necessary, predict how much spare money you will have for leisure, luxuries, and unexpected needs, and plan your spending. Knowing what to expect is one of the best ways to minimize anxiety about retirement.

Retirement savings and expenditure
After retirement your spending habits will undoubtedly change. Anticipating these changes and carrying out sound financial planning can help you maintain a good standard of living. Everyone's spending habits change in different ways. For example, you may save money by not having to travel to work every day, pay for lunch, or socialize after work. However, you may find that you spend more on gas if you use the car more during the day or travel more often to visit relatives. Some of your household bills may also rise because you spend more time at home.

THE EFFECTS OF INFLATION ON YOUR INCOME

A pension that is linked the cost of living index will keep pace with inflation. But for income that is a fixed sum, the effect of inflation—even a modest increase—can have a big impact over a period of years. For example, at an annual inflation rate of 3 percent, the value of a given sum of money will fall to 74.4 percent of its original level in just 10 years; in other words, $1,000 will be worth just $740. This chart shows how the value of money shrinks at different inflation rates. To offset this effect, it is a good idea to put some money in investments that will grow in value.

	ANNUAL INFLATION RATE			
YEARS	3%	5%	7%	10%
5	86.3	78.4	71.3	62.1
10	74.4	61.4	50.8	38.6
15	64.2	48.1	36.2	23.9
20	55.4	37.7	25.8	14.9
25	47.8	29.5	18.4	9.2
30	41.2	23.1	13.1	5.7
35	35.5	18.1	9.4	3.6

CHANGING RELATIONSHIPS

Throughout your time together, you and your partner have no doubt coped with many important life changes, but there will be more to come as you move from middle age into the later years.

Children leaving home and retirement from work can have a big effect on your relationship with your partner and on your emotional needs. The two of you will probably spend more time together than ever, and this can bring difficulties by exposing problems in your relationship that may have remained undetected or ignored for many years. To cope with such lifestyle changes successfully, it is important that you try to understand each other's changing needs, give each other loving emotional support, and be willing to face up to problems and find solutions to them.

Counselors agree that any kind of change is potentially stressful, but as you age, changes can occur with increasing and alarming frequency. Not only are there the physical effects of getting older, but there may be financial, work, or social pressures that put your relationship under stress. This is also a time, however, when you and your partner can reconfirm and improve your relationship and enjoy more leisure time and freedom from the responsibilities of work and raising children.

NEW PRESSURES

The additional time spent together after retirement can place new strains on a relationship, possibly causing resentment and irritation. Often a woman has retired from the workforce earlier or has had extended breaks from outside employment because of child rearing and has already developed an active life outside of work. She may resent the intrusion of her partner into an already busy and fulfilling social life.

To avoid seeing too much of each other and possibly getting on each other's nerves as a result, try to balance time spent together with time spent on your own and on outside interests. It is also useful to agree on how you are going to share your domestic chores, such as cooking, shopping, housework, and gardening.

Some men find leaving their job particularly stressful. Traditionally, men are more focused on their careers as defining their usefulness and status in the world, and retirement can undermine their self-confidence drastically. They may feel insecure and place excessive demands on their partner as a result. For this reason it is essential that both you and your partner recognize the importance of new interests in order to give real meaning and structure to your daily lives. (For ideas on activities in which to become involved, see page 48.)

LEAVING THE PAST BEHIND
A child leaving home can be an opportunity for exploring new directions. A good start might be to redecorate your home, putting now unused rooms to new uses.

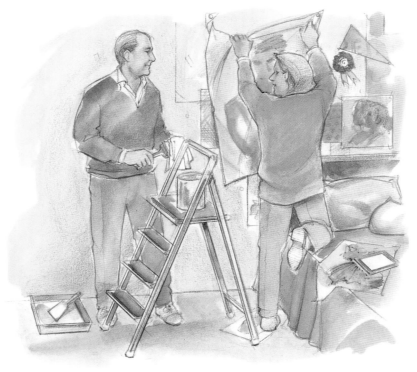

Another possible consequence of retirement is that any long-standing but hidden or ignored difficulties in your relationship can bubble to the surface. During your working years it is often easy to miss the warning signs, especially if both of you have jobs, because your attention is distracted from them. You can do much to avoid this pitfall by maintaining good communication with your partner throughout your relationship so that any problems are identified and dealt with as they arise. Be honest in expressing your feelings, but try to balance this honesty with respect for your partner's views as well as your own.

When you retire, you should talk through the inevitable changes with your partner. If you understand each other's feelings about your new way of life, you will find it easier to deal with the practical and emotional effects. First, consider your own reactions to retirement, such as whether you are looking forward to it or are feeling anxious about it. Think about how the prospect of retirement will affect your self image. If you have any worries or misgivings, you will need your partner's support and encouragement in order to overcome them. Likewise,

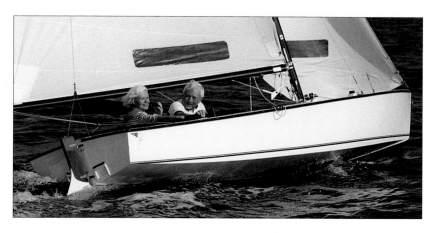

your partner will have his or her own feelings and concerns about the effects of your retirement. You must be prepared to acknowledge these feelings and do whatever is necessary to help him or her adjust to the changing circumstances.

Both of you should be willing to make compromises on practical matters, such as how you will spend your money and where you will live, as well as on the emotional side of your life together. You will need to agree on how you are going to spend your time, both separately and together.

Physical change will also place strain on both partners. Menopause, which typically occurs between the ages of 45 and 55, can be a difficult time for both the woman and her partner. Menopause can bring with it a range of physical and emotional symptoms (see page 68). For example, vaginal dryness and loss of libido can place a strain on a couple's sex life, and in many women mood swings and depression cause emotional distress. Ideally, both partners should take time to become informed about menopause so that its effects can be more readily understood and overcome. Discussing feelings and symptoms should help you and your partner deal better with any problems.

GETTING SUPPORT

If your relationship has generally been smooth and satisfying but suddenly becomes rocked by conflict because of changes such as menopause or retirement, you may need to seek counseling. Your family doctor or a sex therapist can advise you on sexual problems, and you can get help for many other problems from a counselor. The choices of subjects in which counselors specialize can range from relationship and marriage to bereavement and financial matters. To find

WORKING TOGETHER
A sport in which both partners have to work together and trust each other can be very rewarding for all aspects of the relationship.

KEEPING YOUR MARRIAGE ALIVE

A good marriage does not, as a rule, come naturally. It is usually necessary to work at preserving a relationship.

▶ *Set time aside to be with each other every day so that you can share experiences and discuss any problems.*

▶ *Listen to your partner and show that you have heard and understood what he or she has been saying, rather than just waiting for your partner to finish talking so you can begin.*

▶ *Even if you disagree with your partner's point of view, respect his or her opinions and try to see problems from both sides.*

▶ *Be assertive about your feelings and express them to your partner.*

▶ *Don't take your partner for granted; show your appreciation of your relationship on a regular basis.*

▶ *Give each other space, but make sure you do some activities together so you have shared experiences.*

CASE STUDY

A Marriage Under Strain

Couples often undergo a difficult transition period after such a dramatic change as retirement. One retired partner may feel at loose ends, and boredom may make that person overly dependent on the other. If two people do not communicate well with each other, unhappiness and strain within the marriage can result.

Alf, who is 66 and married to Diane, recently retired as the manager of a local travel agency. He devoted a lot of time and energy to his work and had no hobbies or outside interests. As a result, he now feels lost and bored without work to occupy him. He relies on Diane to organize his day and helps her with all the household tasks, such as shopping and cooking. Diane, however, has become increasingly involved in her work as a part-time aide at a local school for the deaf and is beginning to resent the lack of time she now has to herself; she feels that Alf is invading her space. Their marriage is becoming increasingly strained, and their sex life has also suffered, although neither has discussed their feelings.

WHAT SHOULD ALF AND DIANE DO?

Alf and Diane need to discuss their new way of life and how they can better adapt to it. They should consider taking up some joint interests, as well as spending time doing separate activities. Alf has to structure his days so that he is not so dependent on Diane for company. He played golf when he was younger and might think about taking up the sport again. After managing a business, Alf feels wasted without something to organize, so perhaps he could become involved with some committees. Alf and Diane should talk more and try to renew their intimacy with each other in order to boost their sex life.

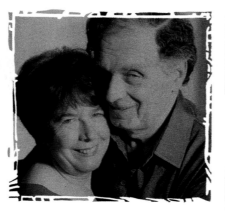

SEX LIFE
Poor communication between partners and resentment of each other can lead to problems in a couple's sex life.

EMOTIONAL HEALTH
Repressing feelings can result in built-up anger and stress.

LIFESTYLE
Lack of direction after retirement can cause depression and frustration for both partners.

Action Plan

SEX LIFE
Spend more time communicating in order to confront and resolve problems. Perhaps try some form of massage to increase physical intimacy and improve sex life.

EMOTIONAL HEALTH
Talk about feelings openly and honestly to resolve underlying tensions. Consider getting some counseling if problems persist.

LIFESTYLE
Look for hobbies and other activities to share and to undertake individually.

HOW THINGS TURNED OUT FOR ALF AND DIANE

Alf joined a golf club and soon was organizing a tournament. The first prize was a holiday weekend, which he arranged through his old firm. The event was a great success, and Alf is now very involved in the club. Alf suggested to Diane that they take up ballroom dancing because they first met each other at a dance. Their dancing evenings, which they enjoy tremendously, have brought them closer together again, fostering renewed intimacy.

a suitable counselor, ask your doctor to refer you to one or contact a national or local organization that offers advice on the kind of problem you are facing. In some cases, such as when a counselor works for a charity or church, counseling will be free, but in others you will have to pay, so find out how much it is likely to cost you and, if necessary, shop around.

If you have managed your whole life without outside help, you may feel that it should not be necessary to seek it now. Yet, as with everything else in life, circumstances change. If you and your partner are embroiled in battles, then it may be wise to seek objective advice, whether it concerns financial or sexual matters or anything else.

SEX IN THE SENIOR YEARS

Many people assume that sexual activity declines or ceases sometime around middle age. This may be true for some individuals and couples, but others find that the older they get, the more they value the closeness and intimacy of sex.

When you are in a long-term relationship, the pattern of your lovemaking matures and its emotional side—the feelings of love, intimacy, trust, and togetherness that it engenders—becomes more important than physical excitement.

In general, your overall level of sexual activity in old age will mirror that of your younger years, and if you have always enjoyed sex, you can continue to do so in your sixties, seventies, and beyond. The frequency of intercourse may decline, perhaps to once or twice a month, but this need not give rise to concern because it may be offset by an increase in other intimate activities, such as kissing and cuddling.

Provided that you and your partner remain in good overall health, you can continue to be sexually active for the rest of your lives, although there are bound to be adjustments in your sex life as you both change physically. Many men take longer to

become aroused, their erections aren't as rigid, and the intensity of their orgasms decreases. They may also take longer to reach orgasm (not always a disadvantage), and afterward may need more time—hours or even days—to get another erection. Their sex drive begins to decline with age.

The frequency and intensity of orgasms also decrease for many women after menopause, usually as a result of hormonal changes. To avoid discomfort during sex, they may have to use some form of lubricant to overcome the vaginal dryness that is common. However, a number of women find that orgasm is easier to reach and happens more frequently. In 1981 the Star-Weiner Report on Sex and Sexuality in the Mature Years noted that in sexually active women, the frequency of orgasm increases in each decade after menopause, up to and including the eighties. Many women feel more sexually liberated when the chances of becoming pregnant and the inconvenience of contraception are no longer considerations.

As you and your partner grow older, you will need to adapt to each other's changing sexual needs. The key to this is communication and understanding. Be honest with each other about your sexual needs and feelings, discuss any anxieties or problems, and try to resolve them sympathetically and constructively. If serious physical or psychological problems arise, don't hesitate to consult your doctor or a relationship counselor. In most cases such problems can be remedied or there will be some way of managing and overcoming any negative effects you may experience.

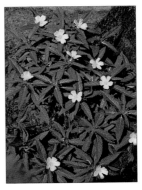

DAMIANA
This Central American herb contains a natural form of the male hormone testosterone and has been used traditionally as a sexual restorative for men. However, no effective uses have been verified by modern science.

TIME FOR SEX
Try making love in the morning or afternoon, when you are less tired and your mind and body are more active.

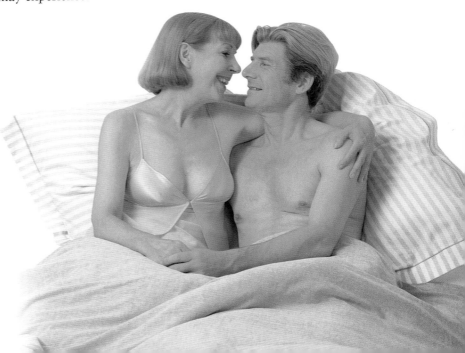

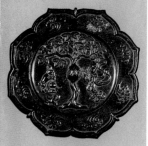

Chang E

The Chinese goddess Chang E was banished from heaven and made a mortal. She and her husband acquired the herb of immortality so that they could return, but there was only enough for one person. Chang E stole the herb and set off for heaven but managed to get only as far as the moon. She is now condemned to live there forever.

MAINTAINING SEXUALITY

Regular sexual activity, whether through intercourse or masturbation, helps reduce the physical effects of aging on your sexual organs in the same way that exercise keeps your muscles firm and strong. It also boosts your sex hormone levels; older men and women who maintain a regular sex life have higher levels of sex hormones and consequently a higher sex drive than those who become sexually inactive.

When you make love, genuine intimacy is more important than performance. Physical arousal may take longer than it did when you were younger, so spend plenty of time on gentle, leisurely foreplay, including manual or oral stimulation. Dedicating this time to each other is a great way to share intimacy with your partner and can be as satisfying and fulfilling as penetrative sex.

You should try to make each other feel attractive and desirable, and neither of you should expect orgasm every time you make love; if it happens, treat it as a bonus. Performance anxiety about achieving and giving orgasm can reduce sex drive and take the enjoyment out of lovemaking. If this is a problem, try taking full intercourse off the agenda for a while and concentrate on showing your affection and desire for each other in other ways. Always remember that making love is not simply a physical activity. It is also a way of creating feelings of intimacy that help you show your continuing love and affection for each other as your relationship matures.

FAMILY RELATIONSHIPS

Your relationship with your partner is bound to be affected by changes within your family. If you have children, you will probably experience mixed emotions when they leave home. You will undoubtedly feel pride in having raised them and in seeing them make their own way in the world and may welcome being free of the responsibility for their day-to-day lives. You might even be glad to have much more time for yourself and your partner, but these positive feelings are likely to be combined with a sense of loss, some sadness, and perhaps even loneliness.

These feelings soon fade, and you will get used to another routine, but you and your partner will need to give each other plenty of emotional support until this happens. Try to remember that this is not the end of your relationship with your children; it is simply a new phase in which you can relate to your child as an adult.

Whatever feelings you and your partner may have about separation from your children, use it as an opportunity to renew your own relationship. Many couples relish the time they have together in this period. It is often the first opportunity they have had to

OVERCOMING THE EMPTY NEST

Some people find it difficult to adjust to their children leaving home. The "empty nest syndrome" can provoke long-lasting sadness and emotional emptiness that can be overwhelming, and it may seem impossible to shake it off. However, there is much you can do to prevent this from happening to you.

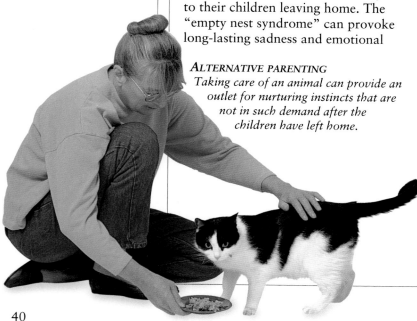

ALTERNATIVE PARENTING
Taking care of an animal can provide an outlet for nurturing instincts that are not in such demand after the children have left home.

▶ *Consider redecorating the children's rooms; don't keep them as a museum to the past. Think about how their rooms might be adapted to your new needs—perhaps as a studio or study.*

▶ *Allow your children their independence but show that you are interested in their lives and proud of their achievements. At the same time, let them know you have your own interests and life to lead.*

▶ *Make a real effort to increase your socializing. Invite friends and neighbors over and make sure that you get out of the house frequently as well.*

spend time alone with each other since they were first married. Their companionship and intimacy deepen, and some say it is almost like a second honeymoon.

Some couples, however, face difficulties when their children leave home. For example, if a woman has devoted all her attention to her children at the expense of her partner's emotional needs, he may have become distanced from her. When the children have gone, it can take a lot of effort from both partners to heal the rift that has developed between them. If this is the case, a relationship counselor may help.

For a relationship to last over decades and provide mutual emotional growth and satisfaction, both people must be good communicators and possess problem-solving skills, and they should share mutual interests. A relationship can survive financial, sexual, or any other problem if both partners are able to express themselves effectively, as well as truly listen to each other. Equally important is the ability to express feelings with assertion, not aggression. Maintaining empathy toward your partner is vital in order to understand how he or she feels.

The key areas in which men and women go adrift are in coping with each other's differences, in resolving disagreements, and in not paying attention to the feelings that go on beneath the surface. Spend as much time as you can trying to resolve problems before giving up on a relationship.

DIVORCE AND REMARRIAGE

The decision to divorce or separate in later life is an extremely difficult one to make. If you have tried to resolve your differences, have seen a counselor, and are still unable to save your marriage, you may have to face up to the pain of a divorce.

In order to cope, try to sort out practical details first. Consider financial arrangements, where you will live, and what your new life will be like. For example, will you have to work to make ends meet? It is often helpful to find a person or support group who can offer advice because divorce is usually an emotionally turbulent time.

You need to think about how divorce will affect your position among your family and friends. Social relationships are bound to change, especially if you have been part of a couple for a long time. Perhaps the biggest hurdle is to face the world as a single person

---

CHECKLIST

If your relationship is going through a bad period, don't give up without trying to save it first.

✔ *Think about your life in general. Is your partner really responsible for your unhappiness or could there be other factors in your life that are upsetting you?*

✔ *Think about the good points of your relationship.*

✔ *Think about your own behavior. Are you being unreasonable or unfair? Is there an issue that is making you unhappy and you have not discussed it with your partner?*

✔ *Make a real effort to talk to your partner about problems or disagreements without being aggressive.*

✔ *Imagine your life alone. Will you really be happier?*

✔ *See a counselor. A third person can often help to put things in better perspective.*

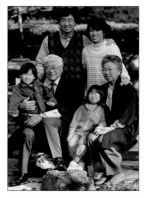

FAMILY SUPPORT
A long partnership will undoubtedly go through rough times. When a relationship between two people becomes difficult, children or grandchildren can sometimes provide a bridge for reestablishing communication.

---

again. Going to social events alone can seem pretty daunting. However, it is vital to overcome these fears; if not, you may be in danger of cutting yourself off and becoming increasingly isolated. Try not to become trapped in negative emotions, such as anger, bitterness, guilt, or a "poor me" attitude after your relationship has ended. Allowing thinking like this to prevail will do you more harm than good.

According to statistics, remarriage in later life is very common. On average, five out of every six divorced men and three out of four divorced women remarry. Most of these marriages are successful because people have learned from mistakes made in former marriages. However, it is helpful to be aware of certain factors. Think about what you expect from marriage. Is companionship enough or do you want a close, intimate relationship? Most experts agree and surveys confirm that it is best to wait at least a year after a divorce before remarrying. This period allows emotional wounds some time to heal and permits an individual to develop a sense of identity once again.

Coping with

Grief

The grieving that follows the death of one's partner is a necessary process that helps a person come to terms with the loss. No one should try to cut grieving short, but there are ways to make it more bearable.

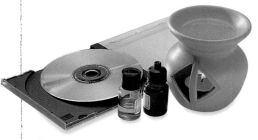

RELAXATION AIDS
Clary sage (Salvia sclarea) essential oil can help release the emotions of grief, and a meditation tape or CD may help you to relax.

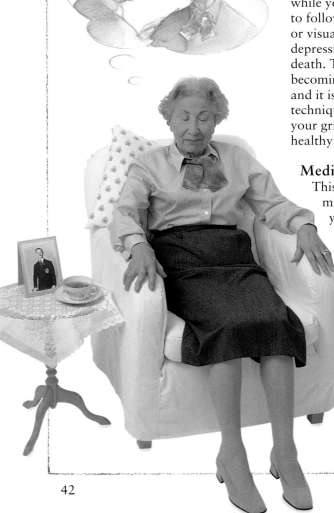

After a death, learning to relax is an important aspect of allowing yourself to grieve. Meditation and visualization can encourage a sense of continuity and acceptance, as well as help to relieve the pain of loss, by focusing your thoughts on your loved one and his or her importance in your life. This process is vital for your well-being.

EFFECTIVE RELAXATION TECHNIQUES

In the early days of bereavement, you might feel like just spending time at home alone with your thoughts. This can be beneficial, but after a while you may find it more helpful to follow a program of meditation or visualization to help heal your depression or anger at your partner's death. There is a very real danger of becoming paralyzed by your grief, and it is easy to do so. The following techniques can help you to relax so your grief can follow a natural and healthy course.

Meditation
This is a way of calming your mind to mentally refresh yourself. It can be a good therapy on its own or can be used as preparation for visualization. You may have to try meditating a number of times before you really feel the benefit, so do not be discouraged if you do not succeed on your first attempt. Find a comfortable position, close

MIND HEALING
Your imagination can allow you to settle any unresolved issues with your late partner.

your eyes, and relax your muscles. Try to empty your mind of thoughts. If it helps, focus on a single object, such as a candle or an ornament. When a thought pops into your mind, gently push it away. Sit quietly like this for 20 to 30 minutes.

Visualization
Visualization involves imagining a scene rather than clearing your mind, and many people find it easier. As for meditation, begin by closing your eyes and relaxing your muscles. If you wish, you can start with a brief session of meditation. Then imagine yourself walking out of the room to a place where your partner is waiting for you. Picture your partner in your mind in as much detail as possible and imagine that you are having a conversation. If it helps, say the words out loud. If there is something you always wanted to say to your partner but never did, find release by talking to him or her now. Say whatever you want to—for instance, tell your partner about your regrets or hopes and, if you have any questions, ask them and let your partner answer. You will probably find this a calming experience, and you can return to talk with your partner any time you choose.

COPING WITH ILLNESS AND DEATH

It can be particularly distressing if your partner falls ill when both of you are getting on in years. You might not have the strength and stamina to provide as much practical help and support as you would like, and the thought that he or she is going to die may never be far from your mind.

At such a time, especially if you are caring for your partner at home, you should try to share the physical and emotional burdens by accepting any offers of help from family, friends, or professional caregivers. If you try to cope alone, your own health may start to suffer and you might become increasingly less able to give your partner the help that he or she needs.

BEREAVEMENT

If the worst happens and you lose your partner, it is important not to suppress or deny the complex mixture of emotions that you will be feeling. For most people the initial reactions to the death of someone dear to them are numbness and disbelief. Grief often does not appear immediately, especially while a person is coping with practical matters, such as informing family and friends of the death and making arrangements for a funeral or memorial service. It may only be later, perhaps after the funeral, that the grieving process begins.

During the grieving process, it is important not to neglect your own needs. Look to your friends and family for support and a shoulder to cry on; they will be glad to help. After the initial shock of your loss, establish and maintain a daily routine so that your practical needs are met. Try to keep busy to avoid brooding and stagnation and make sure you look after your physical, as well as emotional, health. This means eating regularly and well and also continuing to exercise. If it helps to stave off loneliness, try to do some everyday things in the company of others—for example, sharing a meal with friends or relatives. If you have been involved in community organizations, continue these activities.

Do not be afraid to show your grief and don't try to hurry the grieving process; there are a number of emotional stages to go through before you will be able to accept your loss. These stages may include anger at your separation, perhaps feelings of guilt about things you did or did not say or do while your partner was still with you, and fear about your own mortality. These are all normal emotions, so you should not feel selfish or guilty about them. The intensity of these feelings will lessen and eventually they will pass, leaving you more and more with positive feelings and fond memories of your life together.

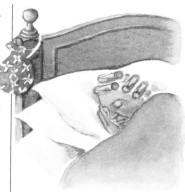

COMFORT BAG
It can be difficult to adjust to sleeping on your own after you have been used to the company of a partner. A simple comfort bag containing sprigs of soothing and soporific herbs, such as chamomile and lavender, can help you have an undisturbed night's rest.

FLOWER REMEDIES TO HELP YOU COPE

Using flower remedies can be helpful in times of emotional upheaval. These were developed in Wales by Dr. Edward Bach in 1929. He believed that the purpose of every person's life was to fulfill his or her individuality but that negative emotional states lie in the way of self-discovery and can lead to illness. He was convinced that nature has the power to heal any ailment—physical or mental—and he used his intuition to discover the healing flower remedies.

To cope with the range of emotions accompanying grief or any other jolting change in life, try the following: willow to help with acceptance; honeysuckle for depression; walnut for change; holly for frustration; Star of Bethlehem for shock; and pine for sleeplessness.

A NATURAL CURE
Add one or two drops of your desired Bach flower remedy to a glass of water. Take the remedy whenever you need it for at least three weeks. Many people find that their state of mind improves rapidly.

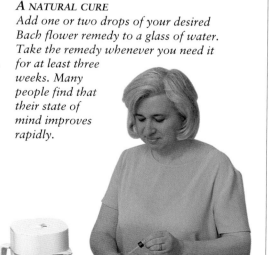

KEYS TO HAPPINESS

A positive attitude, an inquiring mind, an active lifestyle, and plans for the future are important aspects of continuing happiness and contentment as you grow older.

How much you enjoy retirement and old age depends to a great extent on your attitude toward them. If you approach them with gloom and pessimism and expect this period to be one of decline and deterioration, this is probably how it will turn out. Such an outcome would be a terrible waste of what should be a satisfying time of your life, one in which you have the freedom to take up new interests and meet new people. Don't let age defeat you; look at this stage as a time of positive change.

KEEPING A POSITIVE ATTITUDE

Your chances of having a long and happy retirement will be immeasurably increased if you keep a positive attitude toward life. If you expect new and interesting things to happen to you and actively seek them out, the likelihood is that they eventually will.

Learning how to enjoy the present and making the most of each day are useful habits to develop. While there is no harm in taking pride in your past accomplishments,

it is important to continue seeking out the future. Positive words, thoughts, and actions can make you physically and mentally stronger. They must be practiced daily, however, to have a good effect. Making an effort to look on the bright side can pay big dividends. Even though you cannot always prevent negative events, by controlling the way in which you deal with them, you diminish their impact on your life.

GOOD FAMILY RELATIONSHIPS

Maintaining a positive outlook is much easier when you have the support of relatives and friends. Good family and social relationships are important ingredients of a happy life at any age. But when you retire, they can be especially valuable because they give you a sense of belonging and being valued and wanted, feelings that can sometimes be in short supply when you no longer have a job to go to.

You may want to see more of your family when you retire, for example, by visiting them or having them stay with you. If you do not, there is no need to feel guilty about it—you are entitled to decide how you are going to spend your time. If you don't see your family very often, try to keep in regular touch by letter or phone.

One of the benefits of retirement is that it gives you the opportunity to spend more time with your children and grandchildren if you have them, which can be enjoyable and rewarding for all concerned. Spending time with younger family members gives you an opportunity to pass on your parenting skills and to help your children in practical ways, such as by looking after your grandchildren occasionally on weekends and during holidays. You will benefit from

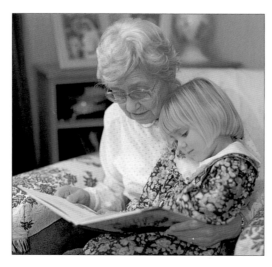

CARING FOR GRANDCHILDREN
Providing a link with past generations and family traditions, grandparents have a vital role to play in the raising of children.

your grandchildren's company and become more involved in their upbringing. And your children will most likely welcome some time to themselves.

There are, however, some pitfalls to avoid. You shouldn't take on more responsibility than you want or can handle, and you must avoid dictating how your children should raise their offspring. If you have any comments to make, be tactful, constructive, and discreet. Never criticize your children's parenting skills in front of their own children because it will cause resentment and could undermine their parental authority as well. Remember also that your children and grandchildren have their own lives to lead, so it may not always be convenient for you to visit them or for them to come see you when you desire it.

THE IMPORTANCE OF FRIENDSHIPS

Many of the greatest pleasures in life stem from close friendships. Indeed, for some people friends can be closer and more supportive than family, especially if relatives live far away. More casual friends and acquaintances also play an important part in adding to the fun in your life.

Friendships, like any other relationships, develop over time. They often start off casually, then gradually deepen, and as they do so, they often seem to become more casual again because old friends trust each other

enough to be less intense. This does not, of course, mean that you can afford to take long-term friends for granted. If you neglect your friends, you risk losing them.

Sometimes friendships end anyway—perhaps because of a serious argument, because one of you moves to another area, or simply because you drift apart or no longer share the same interests. It is important to be able to make new friends (see the box on page 46). Find interests and activities that bring you into contact with new people. Because first impressions can be important, take care of your appearance and develop your social and conversational skills.

Making friends with younger people as well as with those in your own age group has a lot to commend it. You can give them the benefit of your experience and wisdom, and they can bring you new insights and ideas and help you keep in touch with the rapid changes of modern life.

FINDING NEW INTERESTS

The people who get the most out of life are those who put the most into it, and this applies in old age as much as at any other time. If you keep your mind and body active, you will enjoy your retirement more, feel happier and more content, and probably stay healthier and live longer than if you let yourself lapse into inactivity.

Staying active after retirement is not difficult, but it does require some planning. What you should aim for is a mixture of activity and relaxation, home-based activities and outside interests. There is no need to be constantly on the go—being able to slow down is one of the benefits of retirement. Plan your activities so that the pace of your life varies from day to day and from week to week. Making your weekend activities different from those of your weekdays can help you achieve this, and it also gives your life a regular rhythm and pattern that prevents one day from becoming much like the next, which can be depressing.

Because you will be spending more time at home when you retire, it is a good idea to engage in at least one hobby or other activity that you can pursue there. You should also develop outside interests in addition to your home-based activities. This approach has a number of advantages because the range of outside interests available is far greater than the choice

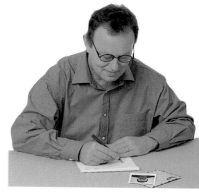

PEN PALS
Keeping in touch with faraway friends brings an awareness that you are connected to other people. Writing and receiving letters or e-mail can be as rewarding as meeting people face to face.

THE GOOD OLD DAYS
Photographs and journals of important events help preserve memories, and leading a full life in the present will ensure that you have plenty to remember in the future.

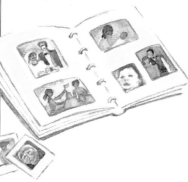

KEEPING FRIENDS

The following guidelines can help you maintain strong friendships:

▶ *Don't take friends for granted. Show them that you value their company.*

▶ *Keep in touch. See your friends regularly; if you can't, then call them or write to them and send cards on special occasions, such as birthdays.*

▶ *Offer advice only if you are asked for it. Respect your friends' privacy and their ability to make their own decisions.*

▶ *Offer help when it is clearly needed, for instance, if they are moving or a partner or other family member is ill.*

▶ *Try not to burden friends with all your own problems. While it's helpful to share worries and doubts, make sure that you share some enjoyable times too.*

MAKING NEW FRIENDS

Friends can be as important as family, especially for people who live far from their relatives. It is always beneficial to make new friends, however active your social life is already. There are many ways to achieve this, and each new person may provide valuable enrichment to your life.

▶ *Be open-minded about the potential for new friends; they can be found in many places, sometimes surprising ones. Be friendly with all the people you encounter, whether they are neighbors or local businesspeople.*

▶ *Work at initiating friendships. Make the first move in inviting someone over. We all fear the possibility of being rejected, but the chances are that if you've started a friendly relationship and shared a laugh, the other person will be delighted to respond.*

▶ *Clubs, classes, and community involvements provide great opportunities to make new friends. For example, communal endeavors—like singing in a chorus, acting in a theater group, or planning a fundraiser for a good cause—are activities that make developing friendships especially easy. Also, taking classes in dancing, painting, or such practical pursuits as woodworking can often break down natural reserves or shyness faster than more formal lecture or discussion groups.*

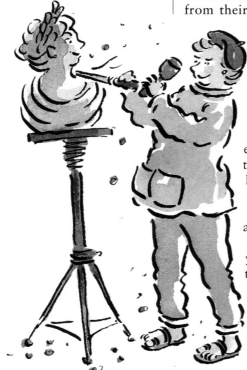

HOME WORK
Taking up an activity that you can do at home can be personally very rewarding. It may even bring financial gain if you have talent and develop sufficient skill.

of home-based activities. Outside interests get you into the company of other people, and some of them provide physical exercise as well as mental stimulation, helping you to keep fit and healthy.

Volunteering

Volunteer work is very popular with retirees, which suggests that many feel strongly that they still have a contribution to make to society. This kind of work can be immensely rewarding, and people sometimes find that they get more satisfaction from their volunteer work than they did from their former paid employment. If doing volunteer work appeals to you, you should have no trouble finding organizations, such as charities or schools, that will be glad for your help. You may, for example, be able to provide real benefit for your community by teaching adult literacy at a local high school or college. Such work is very fulfilling because you can make an enormous difference to another person's quality of life.

Alternatively, you could involve yourself in campaigns to support the interests of wildlife and the environment, in religious activities, or in political activism. Political activism can take a number of forms.

You could, for example, take an active role in campaigning for a candidate; try to get elected to your local governing council or school board; join a lobbying group; or get involved with an international organization like Amnesty International.

NEW SKILLS AND WISDOM

It is never too late to learn something new, and older people are very capable of acquiring new skills and knowledge. In many ways they can be better at it than younger persons because they have a wealth of previous experience to draw on. They may also be more motivated because they are learning through choice and not because they have to. Older persons frequently have more self-discipline as well.

Many people who return to learning in their later years do so to acquire an artistic or practical skill, such as making pottery or doing carpentry. Others simply want to increase their knowledge and broaden their mental horizons. The subjects they study may have little or no practical value for them—they are not training for a job—but studying brings great intellectual stimulation and satisfaction. Many also find that one area of learning leads to another. For example, learning to speak Spanish might encourage someone to study Spanish culture and history as well.

There are many study sources available to you when you retire, whether you want to develop existing skills or knowledge or learn something completely new. For more practical subjects, such as painting, needle craft, or car maintenance, you could try teaching yourself at home, but hands-on instruction in a class is best. Most communities offer a wide range of evening classes at local high schools and colleges, often at nominal fees, and these give you an opportunity to socialize as well as to learn.

You can also study academic subjects at home, either informally by reading books on subjects that interest you, or in a more structured way by taking a correspondence or Internet course. Courses are available for a wide range of subjects and at various levels and usually don't require any prior qualifications. If you want to study a subject in depth, investigate seeking a degree part-time or full-time at a university or college.

Evening classes run by public schools and colleges or by private institutions are another source for academic subjects, as are residential courses for adults run by many colleges and study centers. These courses usually take place during breaks in the academic year, such as summer vacation; by taking a residential course, you can combine your studying with a vacation.

VACATIONS

Taking a vacation at least once a year is just as important after you retire as it was when you were working. It gets you out of your usual routine and surroundings, intro-

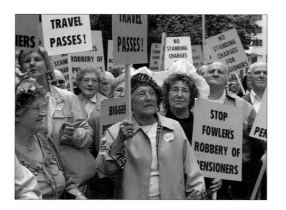

duces you to new places and experiences, and gives you something to look forward to and then back upon. The type and number of vacations you can take will depend on many factors, including your finances, your health, and your personal preferences, but it is worth making the effort to get away now and then, even if only to spend a few days visiting with friends.

One advantage of being retired is that you can take a vacation any time of the year and stay away for as long as you want or can afford. This means that you can visit distant countries that you have always wanted to see and take advantage of out-of-season discounts on travel and accommodations. Many travel operators run tours especially tailored for older people to destinations both local and abroad, often at a discount. These include many types of special-interest

GRAY RIGHTS
Groups that campaign for the rights, concerns, and issues of the elderly have emerged as powerful forces in society. Such organizations as the American Association of Retired Persons and the Gray Panthers in the United States and Canada's Association for the Fifty-Plus have had a number of successes in making life better for older people.

A PURPOSE IN LIFE

There is much evidence that those who continue working or pursuing definite aims in life live longer than those who lack a sense of purpose in their later years. This fact has been graphically illustrated by the lives of many well-known figures. Artists such as Pablo Picasso, Georgia O'Keeffe, Salvador Dali, and Claude Monet lived well into old age and continued to produce highly acclaimed art. Playwright George Bernard Shaw lived and worked until he was 94, when his life ended prematurely following a fall. And eminent physicist Albert Einstein continued working as a university professor and refining his groundbreaking theory of relativity until his death in 1955 at the age of 76.

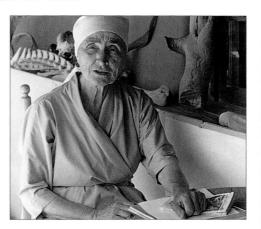

GEORGIA O'KEEFFE
Her painting style developed significantly during her later years. She was still painting at the time of her death at the age of 99.

Expanding Your Horizons with

New activities

*Even if you have always pursued interests outside work,
when you retire, you may have a lot more leisure time to fill.
Don't be reluctant to explore new hobbies and other activities
that will continue to stretch your capabilities and skills.*

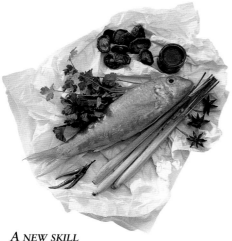

A NEW SKILL
*Different cuisines include ingredients that
you may never have heard of. Learning
how to use unusual foods and making
trips to special shops or supermarkets to
buy them can be as fascinating as the
food preparation itself.*

These days there is an almost endless selection of activities to suit your preferences, abilities, and finances. In making a choice, look for ones that will get you out and about and keep you in the social swim, as well as interests you can follow at home.

Choose activities that you enjoy and find stimulating and that will allow you to develop new skills and abilities rather than simply being a way of passing time. At the same time, avoid hobbies that may take up more time or energy than you

are willing to give because you are unlikely to stick with them.

An easy and relatively inexpensive way to find things to do at home is to take a more creative interest in activities that you would be doing anyway, such as gardening or cooking. Alternatively, you might want to try something that you haven't done before, such as playing a musical instrument. Keep in mind that getting enjoyment from an activity is more important than how skilled you are in its performance.

FULFILLING LEISURE TIME

There are a wealth of activities available to older people wishing to get involved in something new. If you are not sure which one to choose, the chart below may help you decide what would suit you.

DO YOU ENJOY BEING CREATIVE?

Attend an art, woodworking, or pottery class; learn to play a musical instrument; learn to cook an exotic cuisine; do dressmaking or model making; sketch landscapes.

DO YOU ENJOY BEING OUTDOORS?

Take nature walks; go on archaeology digs; do hiking, orienteering, horseback riding, gardening, golf, archery, or lawn bowling.

DO YOU ENJOY A MENTAL CHALLENGE?

Learn to play a musical instrument; join a writers' group; learn a new language; study for a university degree.

DO YOU ENJOY MEETING NEW PEOPLE?

Volunteer at a tourist bureau, museum, or charity shop; join a language conversation class; teach adult literacy; play a team sport.

DO YOU ENJOY CARING FOR OTHERS?

Visit patients in a hospital; help disabled people; be a teacher's aide in an elementary school or play group; care for animals; learn about aromatherapy massage or reflexology.

DO YOU ENJOY ORGANIZING THINGS?

Direct a play for an amateur drama group; organize an outing; arrange trips with a club; form a group of your own choice.

DO YOU ENJOY PERFORMING?

Join an amateur drama group or dance class; join a choir, band, or orchestra; participate in poetry reading groups.

DO YOU ENJOY KEEPING FIT?

Take up a team sport, such as baseball or doubles tennis; learn to ski; take up dancing, aerobics, or jogging.

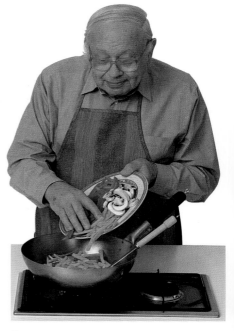

SPICE UP YOUR LIFE
*To prevent cooking from becoming
simply a necessary chore, try experiment-
ing with different and exotic cuisines,
such as Chinese or Thai.*

tours, such as wildlife safaris; archaeological explorations; tours that have a religious, art, or walking focus; and adventure excursions. There is also Elderhostel, which offers inexpensive tours that usually include an educational element.

Whether you plan to travel independently or with a tour group, make sure you will not be taking on more than you can manage; otherwise, your vacation might not be so enjoyable. For example, trying to cope with a tour schedule that is too demanding for you, especially in a hot, humid climate, can quickly tire you out, cause discomfort, and possibly make you ill.

You should also purchase adequate travel insurance, including health coverage, before you leave home. And if you are taking any medication regularly, make sure that you carry an adequate supply with you, especially if you go abroad, where it might be either unobtainable or very expensive.

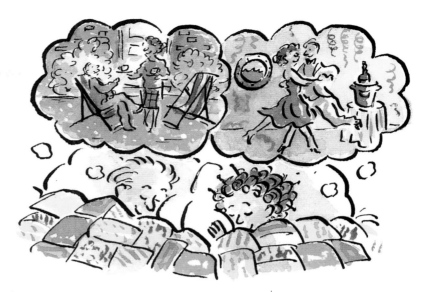

MOVING

For any number of reasons you may choose to move when you retire. For example, if your present home is bigger than you now need because your children have left, moving to a smaller home has many advantages. It will be easier to look after and less expensive to run. Also, if you are renting your present home, the rent for a smaller one will probably be less, depending on its location. If you own your home and sell it to buy a condominium or smaller house, this could give you a useful sum of cash to offset the cost of moving and to spend on vacations and other pleasures or simply to supplement your everyday income.

Another common reason for moving is to settle in a pleasanter area or one with nicer weather, which is why many retired people move from the city to the country, the seacoast, or any place with a warmer climate. You might want to be nearer your children or other relatives or to live in a house without stairs to climb, which can be a problem when you become older.

It is important to plan any move carefully and preferably well in advance so that you can be as certain as possible that your new home will be suitable for your needs and wants. It is easy to concentrate more on the advantages of a potential new home than on possible disadvantages, and the disadvantages may turn out to be more problematic

for you than you had at first thought. For instance, you might miss your friends more than you expected and find it hard to make new ones. Basic amenities such as stores, health care, and leisure facilities might be fewer and farther away, and if you cannot drive or have to give it up for health reasons, public transportation in the area might not be adequate for your needs.

You should also beware of basing your choice of location on misleading impressions; a small village or seaside town might seem an attractive place in which to live when you stay there for a week or two during the summer, butit may turn out to be bleak and empty in winter.

Get as much information as possible about the place in which you plan to settle and perhaps rent a home there for a year to make sure that your choice really is right for you. You will then be able to look forward to spending your retirement in contentment.

Retirement villages

A housing option that has appeal for increasing numbers of older people is a retirement village or complex. These are built to cater specifically to retired people, and they usually contain suitable leisure facilities and other services such as health care.

A well-run retirement village can be an enjoyable place in which to live, and there will usually be an active social scene to help you make new friends. The one drawback is that you might find you miss the company of younger people. If you are considering moving to such a complex, talk to residents about the advantages and disadvantages of

IDEAL RETIREMENT
Communication is vital if you and your partner are going to agree about what type of home and lifestyle you will have after retirement.

BRIGITTE BARDOT
Proving that major changes in lifestyle are possible at any age, French film star Brigitte Bardot gave up her glamorous life to become a prominent campaigner for animal rights issues.

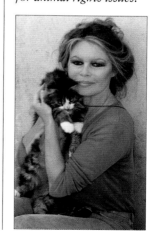

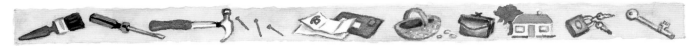

THE PROS AND CONS OF MOVING

Moving means great physical and emotional upheaval and can be an expensive step to take. If you are unsure whether you should take the plunge, try the quiz below.

Answer each question with the letter closest to your situation, add up the number of times you answer a, b, or c, and see the "answers" section at the end.

IN WHAT STATE OF REPAIR IS YOUR CURRENT HOME?

a. It needs a lot of work.
b. It needs a few things done to it.
c. It is in very good repair.

IS YOUR HOME EXPENSIVE TO RUN?

a. It costs a fortune; heat seems to go straight out the roof.
b. It is fairly expensive, but if I am careful, I can manage.
c. My home is well insulated and relatively inexpensive to run.

HOW CONVENIENT ARE LOCAL AMENITIES?

a. If I want to go out shopping, I have to catch a bus and then walk.
b. The stores are a 20-minute walk away, but I often get a ride.
c. I am close to the stores, my doctor, and a community center.

ARE YOU CLOSE TO RELATIVES AND FRIENDS?

a. I feel very isolated. Without the phone I wouldn't speak to anyone.
b. I see relatives now and then.
c. I am good friends with my neighbors and have relatives close by.

CAN YOU GET AROUND EASILY IN YOUR HOME?

a. The stairs are steep and very difficult to manage.
b. The stairs are steep, but I would be able to add a downstairs bathroom if necessary.
c. My home is on one level; it is just the right size and easy to manage.

DO YOU FEEL SECURE IN YOUR HOME?

a. I often worry about security.
b. Sometimes I worry, but I have a strong lock and the outside is well lit.
c. My home feels very secure, and all the neighbors keep an eye out for each other.

ANSWERS

Mostly a: Perhaps your home is no longer suited to your needs. Why not consider a move to a more practical place?

Mostly b: Your home is not ideal in a practical sense. You may want to consider moving or adapting your home to suit you better.

Mostly c: You are happy and secure in your home. Unless you really want to move, there does not seem to be a need to do so.

living there and consider if you would enjoy the prospect. You should also check on what costs you are likely to incur, such as service and repair charges, and make sure that the project is financially secure and well run.

SELF-FULFILLMENT

One secret of happiness in old age is to accept and come to terms with what is, what has been, and what is to come. Life is all about change, and when you recognize the inevitability of aging and accept it, you are much more likely to feel at peace with yourself. Psychologists agree that paying attention to the diversity of your life is an important step toward self-fulfillment.

Strong friendships and family relationships, varied interests, and responsibilities combine to make up a full life. However, you also need time to be alone, to relax, and to take care of your health. A full, varied, and enjoyable life is an insurance policy against the future. If misfortune should befall you, such as losing a friend or suffering an injury, you will still have other activities and concerns to keep you in touch with the world and to help keep you going. Take

pride in your achievements, draw strength and confidence from them, and do not brood on past mistakes. Look toward the future with hope and optimism and seek to enjoy each day to the fullest.

WHAT NOT TO BELIEVE ABOUT OLD AGE

There are myths about old age that can make people unnecessarily worried about their advancing years.

▶ *Old age means loneliness. Actually, older people deal far better with being alone than the inexperienced young, and there are lots of opportunities to socialize.*

▶ *Older people are more vulnerable. In fact, crime against the elderly is rare. For extra assurance, secure your home with adequate door and window locks. You could also take a self-defense class.*

▶ *Money is needed for good health. It is not expensive to maintain a healthy diet and do regular exercise. Visits to a doctor and other health care professionals will not help if you don't look after yourself.*

CHAPTER 3

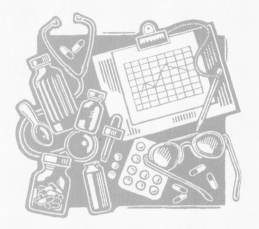

FUNCTIONAL HEALTH

*Many people are concerned about the
increased likelihood of illness and disease
as they grow older. Although ill health may
seem to be unavoidable at times, understanding
how your body works, how it might change, and
the many factors that help prevent disease
can go a long way toward ensuring
good health and peace of mind.*

MAINTAINING GOOD HEALTH

Aging bodies require different medical attention than younger ones. It is especially important in later life to be alert to and understand these changing needs.

Taking responsibility for your health becomes increasingly important as you age. Dealing with preventive measures within your control, such as improving an unhealthy diet and increasing your exercise, can help you avoid many health problems, and regular screening can uncover problems early enough to allow successful treatment.

SCREENING AND HEALTH

Regular screening for certain conditions is generally regarded as good practice for everyone over the age of 50. Most older people should have a checkup once a year, more often if they have a specific problem that has to be kept under observation. The checkup should include certain screening tests, depending on age and sex. These tests may not only detect a disease in its early stages, when it almost always responds more successfully to treatment, but also reveal warning signs of disease, which will allow you to take action to prevent a serious condition from ever developing. In addition, screening helps provide the peace of mind that comes with knowing you are giving yourself the best care possible.

What happens in a screening?

During a typical checkup your doctor will read your blood pressure and order blood tests for cholesterol levels and blood count, and a urinalysis for signs of diabetes.

For women a Pap smear (to look for cervical cancer) is performed routinely, as well as a mammogram (to check for breast cancer), but the frequency varies according to age. After menopause a woman should also have a bone scan to look for signs of osteoporosis. For a man over age 50 an annual prostate exam and a blood test for prostate-specific antigen (PSA) are advised, especially if there has been prostate cancer in the family. For anyone past age 50, flexible sigmoidoscopy or colonoscopy to screen for colon cancer is recommended every five years, oftener if polyps have been found.

If you have particular concerns or a family history of such ailments as heart disease, other tests may also be performed. These include a lung function test for asthmatics; an electrocardiogram (ECG) and possibly an exercise stress test to detect any signs of heart disease; and a chest X-ray, usually given to smokers, who have a high risk of developing lung disease.

CHOOSING A DOCTOR
If you have to choose a new doctor, look for one who is concerned for your overall well-being, keeps convenient hours, is associated with an accredited hospital near your home, and has good backup in case he or she is unavailable. Make sure that you feel comfortable with this person.

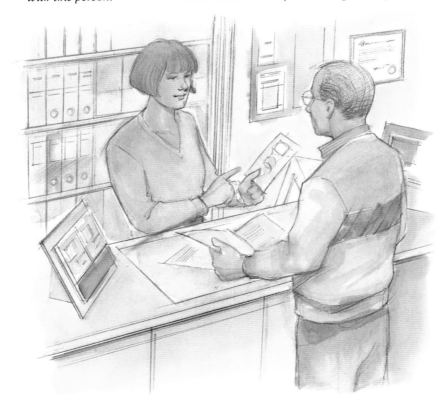

CHOOSING A DOCTOR

Ideally, your doctor should know you and your medical history well, but it is not always possible to remain with the same physician for many years. If you have to choose a new doctor, ask friends for recommendations and perhaps consider looking for a geriatrician, who has special training in the medical problems of older people (see pages 20–21). It is also important to take practical considerations into account. Is the office in a convenient location and do the hours suit you? If the doctor is part of a group practice, ask what other services are available. If possible, visit different practices to find one that best suits you.

If you belong to an HMO in the United States, the doctor you choose must be a member of your plan. Some plans will pay a part of the cost for out-of-system care, but you will end up paying a bigger portion than if you stay within the system. If you are covered by Medicare, you can choose any doctor you want, as long as he or she accepts Medicare patients. In Canada you can select any doctor, but that person does not have to take you if the list is full. If he or she is unable to recommend another doctor, a local hospital or medical society may have lists of physicians who are accepting patients.

Getting the attention you need

Do not be reluctant to ask your doctor questions. He or she should explain fully what is wrong with you and what your options are. If you are not happy with the explanation, consider seeking a second opinion. If your doctor is too busy to discuss things at length with you, ask when would be a convenient time to return.

The more serious a medical problem and its treatment, the more important it is to understand the consequences and make an informed decision. For instance, if you have been told that you need surgery, you should know what the risks are compared to the potential benefits. What is the success rate of this type of surgery? Will it affect your lifestyle? Is there a possibility that you will be disabled in some way? What could happen if you decide not to have the surgery?

ALTERNATIVE THERAPIES

Depending on the nature of your problem, you may opt to seek help from an alternative therapist. Naturopaths, for example,

ALTERNATIVE OPTIONS

If you have a problem that is not life threatening or rapidly getting worse, it may be helpful to consult a complementary practitioner, such as a homeopath or an acupuncturist. This person will usually talk to you at length about your symptoms, giving you the opportunity to review your lifestyle and any beneficial changes you might make. Often doctors don't have time for such individual attention.

deal with a range of problems using a combination of diet, herbs, and sometimes massage to help the body heal itself. They can be particularly helpful if you have digestive problems or allergies. Herbalists and homeopaths also treat a range of problems, including allergies, certain chronic illnesses, and digestive difficulties, without the use of pharmaceuticals that can have unpleasant side effects. Consider seeing a chiropractor for neck and back problems, an acupuncturist or hypnotherapist for relieving chronic pain or overcoming a smoking habit.

Before you visit an alternative practitioner, make sure he or she is registered with a national accreditation body. You should inform both your doctor and your alternative therapist of any treatments you are undergoing so that both can make the best decisions for your health.

WHEN TO SEE A DOCTOR

Consult your doctor if you have a new symptom, a symptom that has persisted for more than two weeks, or a symptom that is steadily worsening. You should also visit your doctor if you have any health concern that is worrying you. Many older people do not see a doctor often enough, and they suffer unnecessary pain and discomfort. Symptoms that demand medical attention include

▶ *Severe chest pain that gets worse with exertion*

▶ *A cough that persists for more than two weeks*

▶ *Hoarseness for more than three weeks*

▶ *Skin ulcers or wounds that won't heal*

▶ *Any new lumps*

▶ *Blood in feces or urine*

▶ *Unusual vaginal discharge*

PREVENTION IS BETTER THAN CURE

Although each system of the body can suffer unique problems, optimum health of all systems generally depends on successful maintenance— that is, on giving your body the right day-to-day care it needs to prevent ill health before it happens or to keep illness from becoming worse if it has already been detected.

While medical science has made great strides over the past century, its power to cure is still limited, and the success of any treatment often depends

on early detection of a disease, as well as your general health.

On the following pages advice is given for dealing with widely different conditions, yet all of it reflects common concerns. Issues of diet, exercise, stress relief, and body awareness come up frequently because they are all involved with enhancing your ability to deal with infection and illness. Natural remedies and alternative therapies that address both body and mind are important to this holistic approach.

Cardiovascular System

Problems with the heart and circulation become increasingly common as people age and can be the source of much distress and anxiety. However, the cardiovascular system responds well to many preventive health measures.

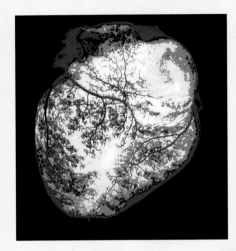

THE HUMAN HEART
Your heart is at the center of your cardiovascular system, pumping blood throughout the body.

THE CARDIOVASCULAR SYSTEM

The cardiovascular system comprises your heart and circulation. Blood moves ceaselessly around the body, carrying life-giving oxygen and nutrients to all the body's cells. It is pumped from the right side of the heart to the lungs, where it takes up oxygen, then returns to the left side of the heart and from there is pumped to the rest of the body.

KEYS TO HEALTH

▶ Cut down on saturated fats in your diet and increase intake of soluble fiber.

▶ Increase your intake of antioxidants (see page 86).

▶ Increase your intake of garlic, ginger, and onions.

▶ Do not smoke.

▶ If you drink, limit your intake to 175 to 200 ml (4 to 5 oz) of wine, 500 ml (12 oz) of beer, or 30 ml (1½ oz) of spirits a day.

▶ Exercise regularly (see Chapter 5).

▶ Have regular medical checkups.

CARDIOVASCULAR HEALTH

Over time the heart and circulation become less efficient. Even a healthy heart muscle slows down; typically, that of a healthy 80-year-old functions at only three-quarters of the speed of one belonging to a healthy 30-year-old. A common problem with the heart that often appears with advancing age is an irregular heartbeat. This can occur for a number of reasons and is alarming but rarely serious. If an irregular heartbeat interferes with a person's everyday life, it can be corrected with a pacemaker.

A good diet can help improve and maintain cardiovascular fitness. This includes limiting saturated fat to 10 percent or less of daily calorie intake because saturated fat can cause the body to produce too much cholesterol. While cholesterol is vital to several bodily processes, too much is implicated in the buildup of fatty deposits that clog arteries. Cholesterol consists of two principal types: high-density lipoprotein (HDL), also

known as "good" cholesterol, and low-density lipoprotein (LDL), known as "bad" cholesterol. The latter is responsible for fat deposits.

To keep cholesterol levels low, it is essential to include plenty of fiber in the diet, especially the soluble fiber found in oat and rice bran, fruits, nuts, legumes, and many vegetables, and to get sufficient exercise.

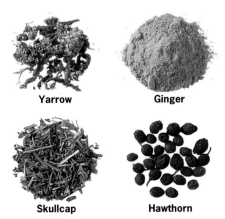

Yarrow

Ginger

Skullcap

Hawthorn

HERBAL CARDIOVASCULAR HELP
Some herbs have positive effects on the cardiovascular system. Taken with the advice of an herbalist and the approval of your doctor, they can help in the management of certain problems. Skullcap, hawthorn, and ginger may help lower blood pressure. Yarrow has a mild vasodilating effect that may improve circulation.

Exercise also increases the amount of oxygen transported to your heart and makes it more efficient. After activity your resting pulse will be slower because more blood is pumped with each beat and with less effort by the heart. This lowers your risk of stroke, heart disease, and other circulatory disorders. (Advice about exercising and its benefits is included in Chapter 5.)

If you already have a heart or circulation problem, such as angina or high blood pressure, exercise will still be of benefit, but it is vital to consult your doctor before embarking on a program. You should start with a gentle form of exercise, like walking, and continue until you are just out of breath but not overtired or in pain. If you have a severe condition, even walking across a room will provide some benefit; it is vital to keep active.

CHELATION THERAPY

Chelation therapy, developed originally to remove toxic metals like lead from the body, is being used by some doctors today to treat cardiovascular problems. It involves flushing the circulatory system with a chelating agent—the chemical ethylenediaminetetraacetic acid (EDTA)—and therapeutic doses of vitamins and minerals to clear fatty deposits from the arteries and veins. The EDTA infusion is administered through a slow drip. Supporters claim that the therapy safely and noninvasively reverses years of damage, but the American Heart Association and other medical organizations say there is insufficient proof as yet of its efficacy.

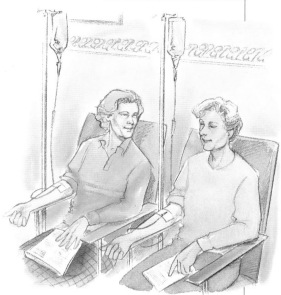

CHELATION TREATMENT
Chelating agents are administered intravenously. An average of 30 treatments is given, each one lasting 3 to 4 hours.

ANGINA

As people grow older, the arteries and veins in the body become less flexible and may also become clogged with fatty deposits. These deposits restrict the flow of blood and increase its pressure in the body. Over time reduced blood flow to the heart will deprive it of vital oxygen, which causes a painful condition called angina. The symptoms themselves are not life threatening,

but the pain can be very frightening. Sometimes it can be difficult to distinguish angina from severe indigestion. If the condition is left unchecked, restriction of the blood flow to the heart can cause permanent damage, even a heart attack. Treatment usually involves prescription drugs, but it is far better to prevent angina through a good diet and regular aerobic exercise.

GARLIC FOR THE HEART

Garlic can be useful in managing cardiovascular disease because it lowers blood pressure and the overall cholesterol level while raising the HDL level. It also helps prevent blood clots that can lead to heart attack. Garlic causes bad breath, however, and in some people, indigestion. Cooking reduces garlic's odor but also destroys some of its active ingredients; raw garlic is best. To offset the odor from raw garlic, you can chew fenugreek or fennel seeds or fresh parsley. Garlic pills produce no odor but should have a coating because stomach acid destroys one of garlic's active ingredients, alliin.

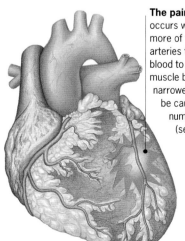

The pain of angina occurs when one or more of the coronary arteries that supply blood to the heart muscle become narrowed. This can be caused by a number of factors (see right).

An atheroma, a fatty substance that can build up on the walls of the arteries, restricts the flow of blood.

A blood clot forms when passing blood cells adhere to the sticky surface of an atheroma.

Spasm, which restricts the blood supply, occurs when an artery or vein has lost its flexibility.

CAUSES OF ANGINA
The blood supply to the heart can be limited by blockages or spasms in the arteries and veins. These can be caused by aging and the gradual deposit of fat on the lining of the arteries. Fatty build-up is caused mainly by a diet high in saturated fat and lack of regular exercise.

BLOOD PRESSURE

Blood pressure, the force at which blood is pumped through the body's arteries, tends to rise somewhat with age as the arteries gradually harden. It also increases under conditions of stress and intense emotion. High blood pressure (a reading of 140/90 or above), also called hypertension, is dangerous because it can lead to such serious conditions as kidney failure, stroke, and heart disease. Symptoms are rare until an advanced stage is reached, at which time they may include light-headedness, headache, and a rapid heartbeat. Once detected, high blood pressure can be controlled through dietary measures and regular exercise, as well as drugs if necessary.

Traditional Chinese medicine uses such herbs as chrysanthemum, peony root, and astralagus to treat high blood pressure. (Low blood pressure is less common and rarely requires treatment.) Western herbalists recommend dandelion and fennel tea and hawthorn or ginkgo biloba extract. Aromatherapists advise adding drops of lavender, lemon, clary sage, or ylang-ylang essential oil to a massage oil or a bath.

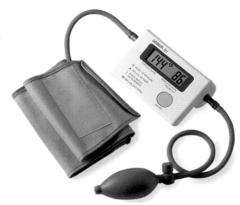

BLOOD PRESSURE GAUGE
If you have a problem with hypertension, it may be a good idea to monitor yourself regularly with a blood pressure gauge that can be used at home.

STRESS REDUCERS

Stress is a fact of everyday life. It is important to deal with stress effectively, especially if you are at risk for heart disease or circulatory problems, because prolonged excess stress makes the blood stickier and thus more likely to clot. Staying physically fit through regular exercise and a healthy diet seems to enable people to cope better with stress; so do relaxation techniques, such as meditation and visualization. Yoga is also an effective stress reducer.

STROKE

Problems arise when blood flow is restricted in any part of the body. The most serious of these is a stroke, which occurs when not enough blood reaches the brain, either because of a blood clot (called a thrombosis) or a narrowed blood vessel. Some strokes are also caused by bleeding in the brain. When the blood supply to an area of the brain is interrupted, the cells there die.

Although strokes can be life threatening and debilitating, many people recover almost completely. Treatments for stroke attempt to restore circulatory health and guard against further strokes—many people have a series of strokes, with the initial one acting as a warning— while preventing muscle wastage and encouraging flexibility.

In addition to physical therapy, some alternative treatments can help with recovery. Acupuncture may be used to treat paralysis caused by stroke, and massage, chiropractic, yoga, and osteopathy can aid in restoring body flexibility and muscle tone, as well as help sufferers to regain greater freedom of movement.

To regulate and improve blood supply to affected areas, homeopaths recommend Arnica 6c and biochemic tissue salt Kali mur. Traditional Chinese medicine uses lovage tuber.

The same dietary and exercise measures that protect your heart and cardiovascular health will also help guard against strokes.

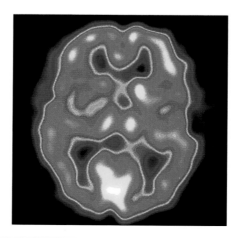

STROKE RECOVERY

Although strokes are rightly viewed as one of the most serious health problems of old age, the outlook for stroke sufferers is not as bleak as you might imagine. Strokes can vary greatly in severity, and only the worst are truly disabling. Even when the damage is considerable, the human brain has remarkable powers of recovery because of a property that neurobiologists refer to as plasticity This enables the brain to find new ways of performing stroke-impaired functions, by circumventing the damaged areas and using parts of the brain that are not normally associated with these functions.

WINDOW ON THE MIND
Modern brain imaging techniques, such as magnetic resonance imaging (MRI), can show which parts of the brain have been damaged by a stroke, helping therapists to target rehabilitation methods.

ANEMIA

There are many types of anemia, all marked by abnormalities in the red blood cells. All types are characterized by fatigue, dizziness, pale skin, shortness of breath, and palpitations.

Iron deficiency anemia, in which the body lacks sufficient iron to make enough hemoglobin—a substance in the blood that carries and delivers oxygen to the cells—is the most common form. It may result from malnutrition, illness, or excessive blood loss—for instance, from a peptic ulcer, heavy menstrual bleeding, or an injury. Sufferers have to make sure they get enough iron (see box, far right).

There are two forms of iron: heme and nonheme. Animal foods contain heme iron, which is the most easily absorbed. Plant foods yield nonheme iron, which is less eaily absorbed,

but its absorption can be enhanced by the presence of vitamin C. Tea, coffee, antacids, and the phytates found in whole grains can interfere with the amount of iron absorbed; they should be avoided in the same meal with iron-rich foods.

Whole foods are always a better source of nutrients than supplements. However, if your diet is not providing enough iron, a doctor or dietitian may advise supplements. You should not take them on your own because they can be dangerous in high doses and a buildup of excess iron can damage the heart.

Two other types of anemia—pernicious (deficiency of vitamin B_{12}) and folic acid (folate) deficiency—are caused by poor nutrition. Meat is a good source of both nutrients; fruits and vegetables are also rich in folate.

GETTING ENOUGH IRON

As people age, they become more vulnerable to mineral and vitamin deficiencies for several reasons, including loss of appetite and a diminished ability to digest food. One important mineral they may lack is iron, an essential component of hemoglobin—the oxygen-carrying protein in blood. Iron-rich foods include

► Liver

► Red meat and chicken

► Seafood

► Spinach and other leafy greens

► Whole-grain and enriched bread and cereals

► Nuts

► Dried beans and other legumes

► Dried fruits

CIRCULATION PROBLEMS

As the cardiovascular system ages, the heart becomes less efficient and the arteries often get narrower; these conditions have an impact on circulation. Poor circulation most often affects the areas farthest from the heart—a condition known as peripheral ischemia. It can be a sign of diabetes (see page 77), but the most common cause is smoking.

Symptoms of poor circulation include cold hands and feet, muscle cramps, and in extreme cases, gangrene in tissues to which the blood supply has been cut off. When circulation to the legs is impaired as a result of atherosclerosis, intermittent claudication (lameness) may occur; the sufferer cannot walk without pain and must frequently pause for rest. This condition is also commonly associated with smoking.

A much more common circulation problem is varicose veins. This condition arises when the valves in veins fail to work properly to push the blood back to the heart, causing

an area, usually in the legs, to swell. If you have varicose veins, try not to stand for long periods, don't cross your legs when sitting, and wear support stockings if necessary.

Ginkgo biloba extract, available from most drug and health food stores, increases circulation to the extremities. Increasing your intake of EFAs (see page 82) may also help.

NETTLE AND HORSETAIL RUB FOR VARICOSE VEINS

Varicose veins can cause aching, tired legs and sometimes skin rashes or ulcers; they are often unsightly as well. Gently rubbing this lotion daily onto the area can help improve the circulation.

1 *Pack 2 handfuls of nettles and two horsetail stems into a sterilized screw-top jar and add 300 ml (10 fl oz) of almond oil.*

2 *After about 12 hours, strain the oil into a sterilized dark-glass bottle. Seal the bottle and keep it in a slightly warm place for three weeks, shaking it every day. The lotion is then ready to apply.*

Respiratory System

Problems with breathing gradually become more pronounced as you grow older. If you take good care of your lungs now, you can improve their capacity and resistance to disease in the future.

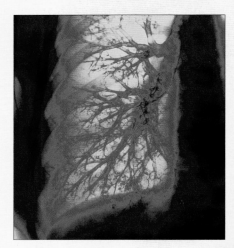

INSIDE THE LUNGS
The lungs contain many branches of bronchioles, here seen as red twiglike shapes in the lung. These supply air to the sacs that feed the blood supply.

RESPIRATORY HEALTH

As we breathe, oxygen is taken into the lungs and carbon dioxide is exhaled. When we inhale, air flows through the mouth and nose down into a tube called the trachea. This eventually divides into millions of tubes known as bronchioles to create an inverted treelike system within the lungs. At the end of each bronchiole are the alveoli, or air sacs. It is through the thin walls of the alveoli that oxygen and carbon dioxide diffuse into or out of the blood. Healthy lungs contain about 300 million alveoli each. Over time the number of alveoli remains the same, but the structure of the lungs and the way they work alters.

KEYS TO HEALTH

▶ Exercise regularly to improve blood flow to the lungs and increase their elasticity.

▶ Do not smoke and try to avoid smoky environments.

▶ Avoid inhaling hazardous chemicals.

▶ Maintain a normal weight.

▶ Maintain a healthy diet (see Chapter 4).

THE EFFECTS OF AGING

Over time the lungs become less efficient. The chest wall—made up of the ribs, the sternum, and the spine—becomes stiffer; the alveoli—tiny air sacs in the lungs—shrink slightly, so they cannot work as efficiently as they once did; and the walls of the lungs become less elastic, reducing the volume of air they can take in with each breath. These changes can cause problems because all the stale air is not expelled from the lungs, and the blood may become starved of oxygen. This is one reason that older people cannot perform as much physical exercise as when they were younger and they are more breathless afterward. The lungs have good reserve capacity, however, and serious breathing difficulties rarely occur unless the lungs are attacked by infection or disease or become incapacitated from smoking or constant exposure to air pollution.

The lungs' defense mechanisms against pollution and germs also become weaker with age. This is why chest infections are a common problem among older people. Because of their lowered immunity and poorer lung defenses, a simple cold can lead to something serious like pneumonia, and problems with the heart can cause fluid to build up in the lungs.

Continuing to stay fit in your later years is by far the best way to protect yourself from lung disease. Adopt a healthy way of eating as described in Chapter 4 and lose weight if you need to (see Chapter 7), so that extra strain is not placed on your lungs. And exercise regularly; vigorous activity increases the elasticity of the lungs, thus counteracting the natural stiffening that gradually occurs with age.

Another way of exercising your lungs is to sing or play a wind instrument. For both these activities you have to use your lungs properly, breathing from the diaphragm and in turn improving lung capacity and strength. Deep breathing is also an important part of yoga exercises.

The lungs are under constant assault from pollutants—from the environment and from smoking or inhaling hazardous chemicals. Exposure to air pollution leads to excessive mucus production, loss of elasticity, tissue inflammation, and destruction of the alveoli. Exposure over a long period may even lead to cancer. Avoiding such irritants will help to keep your lungs healthy.

WARNING SIGNS

See your doctor immediately if you suffer from any of the following symptoms, especially if they are coupled with bouts of drowsiness and confusion.

▶ Sudden worsening of breathlessness

▶ Inability to speak or finish sentences due to breathlessness

▶ Coughing blood or blood-stained sputum

▶ Sudden severe chest pain

COUGHS, COLDS, AND INFLUENZA

A common threat to the respiratory health of older people is a cough or cold that lingers and becomes chronic. The viruses that cause these problems can be extremely virulent, and the elderly and infirm are very susceptible to them. Lung complaints can become serious if minor chest infections are not treated right away. Infection can take hold when the body's immune system is weak and can lead to more serious diseases, such as pneumonia, bronchitis, and emphysema. It is very important to consult your doctor if a chest infection does not clear up quickly.

To ensure a healthy immune system, take special care with your diet, eating regular, balanced meals that include a high intake of fruits and vegetables. Also set aside time for relaxation on a regular basis to mitigate the effects of stress. Stress has been shown to reduce the effectiveness of the immune system.

An even greater threat to health is posed by influenza. The symptoms of flu can cause many related problems for the elderly. Aching muscles can greatly inhibit movement, while fever and vomiting can cause problems with hypothermia (see page 78) and dehydration (see page 80). Proper care is vital when suffering or recuperating from influenza. Remember also that annual vaccinations against influenza are available from your doctor and are recommended especially for older patients as a preventive measure.

FLU RELIEF

Certain herbal teas, which can easily be prepared at home, are useful for relieving the symptoms of colds and flu. (Use 1 to 3 tsp dried herb per cup of hot water and steep for 5 to 10 minutes.) Some herbal extracts are also helpful.

► Gargling with sage or peppermint tea eases sore throat pain.

► Slippery elm lozenges and tea also soothe a sore throat.

► Echinacea (extract capsules or tincture in water 4 times a day) relieves the duration and severity of flu and cold symptoms.

► Eucalyptus (4 drops of oil in a bowl of steaming water) relieves stuffiness and suppresses a cough.

ASTHMA IN LATER LIFE

People who have not suffered from asthma since they were children or who have never had an asthma attack in their lives may be surprised to develop the condition late in life. Asthma can be brought on by the recurrence of a childhood disease or a new allergic reaction, both of which are more likely to occur if the lungs have been weakened by age, illness, or a lifetime smoking habit.

Asthma is usually treated with drugs that relax and open up the airways to relieve the characteristic wheezing. Such drugs also reduce the production of mucus, which can clog the airways. Avoiding dairy products can also be beneficial because these increase the amount of mucus produced. Soybeans and other legumes, dark leafy greens, almonds, and foods fortified with calcium should be substituted to ensure adequate calcium intake.

It can be difficult and distressing to

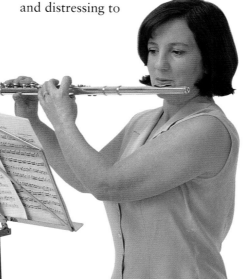

BLOW HARD
Playing a wind instrument, like the recorder, flute, or tuba, is an excellent way to improve lung capacity. Such an activity is particularly beneficial in younger life because the health benefits you gain will stay with you in later years.

ASTHMA ATTACK

Suddenly having trouble catching your breath can be distressing, but it is important to stay calm. Find a place to sit and lean forward with your elbows on your knees. This position elevates the diaphragm and should make breathing easier. Breathe deeply and slowly and try not to panic. Avoid the urge to take shallow breaths, and use your diaphragm to help you breathe more efficiently.

cope with lung problems; it is better to prevent these illnesses by making sure your lungs remain in optimum health. You can mprove the strength and capacity of your lungs by taking preventive measures, such as giving up smoking and exercising regularly. Therapies like yoga and t'ai chi, which incorporate deep breathing in their practice, also help to improve lung capacity. Remember, however, that asthma is a serious condition and requires medical supervision and monitoring to ensure that you are receiving proper treatment.

Digestive System

A common source of problems for older people, the digestive system needs good care because proper absorption of nutrients underpins general health and resistance to many diseases. Learn all you can about what, when, and how you should eat.

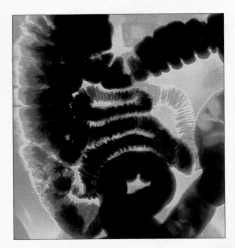

THE INTESTINES
The digestive system includes the large and small intestines, shown above. The large intestine, or colon, absorbs water from digested food and passes the dehydrated matter toward the rectum to be excreted.

DIGESTIVE HEALTH
The digestive system is complicated and finely balanced to enable the efficient conversion of food to meet energy and nutritional needs. The mouth begins this process, breaking up food and moistening it with saliva and digestive enzymes. Food is treated with more digestive enzymes in the stomach and small intestine and is then absorbed; excess water is removed and waste excreted.

KEYS TO HEALTH
▶ Maintain a balanced diet—one that is low in fat and high in fiber and nutrients.

▶ Eat meals regularly; this helps prevent unhealthful snacking and overeating and also promotes regular bowel habits.

▶ Don't skip meals; you can lose out on important nutrients, depress your energy levels, and upset your digestion.

▶ As much as possible, eat fresh rather than processed foods and include plenty of fruits and vegetables.

THE EFFECTS OF AGING

The digestive tract is perfectly capable of working well the whole of our lives, but certain changes occur with age that can affect its efficiency and cause a great deal of discomfort.

As we age, our body tissues become less elastic and start to sag. Common effects of sagging tissues on the digestive system are hiatal hernia and diverticulosis. A hiatal hernia is one in which the muscles supporting the stomach weaken and part of the stomach protrudes up into the chest. It is estimated that as many as 60 percent of people over age the age of 60 have a hiatal hernia. For most of them it makes little difference to the functioning of their digestive system, but it is often the cause of painful heartburn and excessive belching.

Diverticulosis occurs when the support of the colon walls begins to sag and small pockets form in the walls. Waste matter can build up in these pockets and cause diverticulitis, a painful inflammation. Insoluble fiber helps guard against this condition because it is indigestible and exercises and tones the muscles of the system in the process of

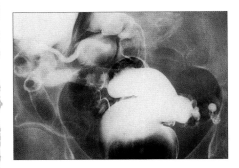

DIVERTICULOSIS
This X-ray shows where the intestinal wall has ballooned out, trapping partly digested food, which then ferments and produces painful bloating.

FOOD ALLERGY

Allergists suspect that many digestive complaints may be due to food sensitivity. If you notice warning signs like these, consider consulting an allergist:

▶ Chronic, recurring digestive difficulties for which a doctor can find no cause

▶ Some apparently unrelated symptoms, for example, a skin rash accompanied by diarrhea

▶ Either a marked craving for or aversion to a particular food

excreting it. Diverticulosis is very common in the Western world but is almost unheard of in African countries, where the diet is largely made up of fiber-rich foods, such as whole grains, fruits, and vegetables.

Hemorrhoids, or piles—swollen veins in the lining of the anus—are a common complaint among older people and are usually a discomfort rather than a serious health risk. However, there is a possibility that they may become infected or extremely uncomfortable. If this should happen, they can be removed surgically. Hemorrhoids can be caused by a diet lacking in fiber, so making adjustments to your diet should help prevent their occurrence.

KEEPING THE DIGESTIVE SYSTEM HEALTHY

Not surprisingly, diet has a huge effect on the health and efficiency of the digestive tract. Insoluble fiber is particularly important for preserving gut muscle tone and promoting regular bowel movement.

Avoiding caffeine and eating smaller portions of food can help reduce heartburn, as can limiting fatty and acidic foods. Simple measures, such as losing weight, reducing alcohol intake, and stopping smoking, together with taking acid-lowering medications can also have beneficial effects. If heartburn is particularly bad at night, try sleeping with your head raised. Drinking plenty of fluids and exercising regularly can also help relieve the pain of heartburn.

Decayed or worn teeth or poorly fitting dentures can also contribute to digestive problems. When food is not chewed properly before swallowing, it is harder to digest. This may prevent the full amount of nutrients from being extracted by the gut.

In some people the secretion of digestive enzymes decreases with age. This reduces the body's capacity to absorb certain nutrients. The result can be malnutrition and must be medically treated. Also with advancing age the stomach produces less hydrochloric acid, which has an effect on digestion.

LIVE YOGURT

Live bacteria in yogurt discourage harmful bacteria and yeasts, such as Candida albicans, *from proliferating in the gut. Eating yogurt with live cultures can also prevent bowel infection and help relieve gastrointestinal disorders, irritable bowel syndrome, diarrhea, and constipation. Some researchers are studying the possibility that it also reduces the risk of bowel cancer.*

THE DIGESTIVE SYSTEM
If any part of the digestive system is damaged or malfunctions, not only digestion but the whole body may suffer.

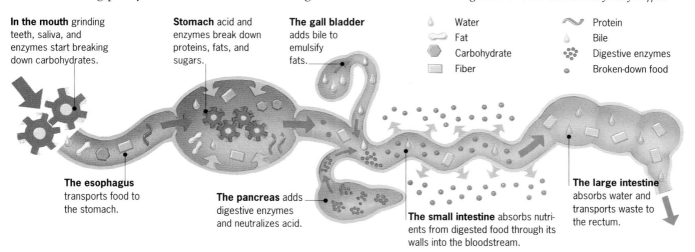

In the mouth grinding teeth, saliva, and enzymes start breaking down carbohydrates.

Stomach acid and enzymes break down proteins, fats, and sugars.

The gall bladder adds bile to emulsify fats.

- Water
- Fat
- Carbohydrate
- Fiber
- Protein
- Bile
- Digestive enzymes
- Broken-down food

The esophagus transports food to the stomach.

The pancreas adds digestive enzymes and neutralizes acid.

The small intestine absorbs nutrients from digested food through its walls into the bloodstream.

The large intestine absorbs water and transports waste to the rectum.

LIFESTYLE FACTORS

Regular exercise increases the blood flow to the digestive system, enabling the muscles to work more efficiently and nutrients to be absorbed more effectively. Aerobic exercise also increases your appetite to healthy levels and burns off fat. However, you should not exercise immediately after eating; your body will not be able to digest your food properly and you may get cramps and indigestion.

Learning how to deal with stress is another step you can take to avoid discomfort with the digestive system. Phrases like "butterflies in my stomach" and problems being felt in the "pit of the stomach" indicate how digestion often reflects and is affected by mood.

Anxiety often manifests itself as diarrhea or stomachache, and worry commonly sends people reaching for alcohol or "comfort foods," which may cause more problems.

Dealing with stress in constructive ways, such as through meditation or visualization (see pages 42 and 132), can reduce unnecessary strain on the digestive system and provide you with other health benefits as well.

HERBAL REMEDIES

A host of herbs can soothe an upset stomach and disturbed digestion. These include

▶ Ginger tea, candied ginger, or chamomile tea to relieve nausea

▶ Anise, dill, or fennel seed tea or peppermint leaf tea to relieve gas

▶ Yarrow leaf tea to relieve bloating, diarrhea, and cramps

▶ Papaya tablets or cayenne pepper to stimulate digestion

▶ Cinnamon to stimulate appetite

Musculoskeletal System

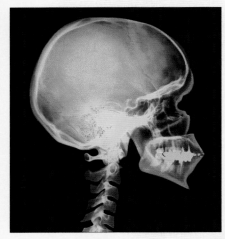

THE SKELETON
The human skeleton is made up of many types of bones and joints. This X-ray of a human skull shows differences in the density and form of bones in the cranium, jaw, and neck.

MUSCULOSKELETAL HEALTH

Bones support the body's internal organs and provide a rigid structure for the muscles to work against. They also accommodate an easily accessible store of minerals. Bones grow most rapidly during childhood and adolescence. However, throughout life they never stop changing and redeveloping, even in old age. Approximately every 200 days new bone is formed by cells known as osteoblasts and old bone is absorbed by large cells known as osteoclasts.

KEYS TO HEALTH

▶ Regularly do weight-bearing exercise, such as walking, jogging, or tennis, to promote and maintain bone strength.

▶ Do stretching exercises regularly to promote and maintain joint flexibility.

▶ Make sure your diet is rich in calcium, magnesium, phosphorus, and vitamin D.

▶ Lose excess weight; being too heavy puts strain on the back and joints, increasing the risk of arthritis.

▶ Do not smoke.

The health of your muscles and bones can have a profound effect on how you cope with aging. Your mobility and independence later in life can be greatly influenced by actions you take today.

THE EFFECTS OF AGING

Bones become less dense and more brittle with increasing age because calcium is lost. From the midtwenties onward, an average of 1 percent of the total bone mass is lost every year. This makes people more prone to fractures, particularly of the hip and wrist, as they grow older. Loss of height and compression fractures of the spine are also common. A decrease in the production of synovial fluid and thinning of the hyaline cartilage, both of which cushion the joints, and the shortening of ligaments can lead to loss of flexibility as well.

Bones are not solid but are made up of a honeycomb of cells. Osteoporosis, the bone-thinning disease, occurs when the holes in bones become larger, making the whole supporting structure thinner and weaker. This is particularly common in postmenopausal women because

OSTEOPOROSIS

Although osteoporosis is more common in women, men can suffer from it too. Almost 1 in 4 women and 1 in 12 men who reach old age will have broken at least one bone. A bone density scan can detect osteoporosis.

the decline in estrogen production seems to accelerate the rate of bone loss. Before menopause the average annual loss of bone mass is as low as 0.3 percent, but this figure increases to up to 3 percent around the time of menopause and remains so for some years afterward. Up to half of North American women over age 45 have some degree of osteoporosis.

Regular weight-bearing exercise, at least one hour three times a week, is a very important factor in maintaining bone density as you age.

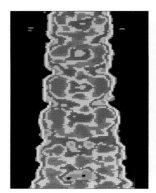

NORMAL BONE
The honeycomb of healthy bone is rigid yet light and strong.

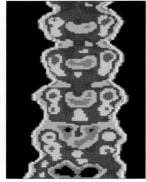

SUBNORMAL BONE
When bone is lost faster than it is replaced, the structure becomes ragged.

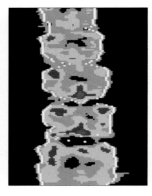

OSTEOPOROTIC BONE
Riddled with holes, this bone is weak, brittle, and easily broken.

DIET AND MUSCULOSKELETAL HEALTH

If you regularly have an adequate amount of calcium, you may prevent many bone problems from occurring in later years. Your daily intake should be at least 800 mg (some experts recommend between 1,000 and 1,500 mg after menopause).

Low-fat and nonfat dairy products are the best sources of calcium. Whole-milk dairy products should be limited because of their high cholesterol and saturated fat content, which can damage the heart. Other good sources of calcium include leafy green vegetables, such as spinach and kale, canned fish with bones, and soy milk, orange juice, and other products fortified with calcium.

Vitamin D is also essential to musculoskeletal health because it aids in the absorption of calcium. Vitamin D is found in fortified cereals, soy products, and milk; egg yolks; and saltwater fish. It is also made in the body on exposure to sunlight.

Magnesium, vitamin K, and boron also play important roles in bone health. A diet rich in fruits and leafy greens should provide adequate amounts of all these nutrients.

WHAT TO AVOID

Several things can interfere with the absorption of calcium or cause it to be excreted in large amounts. These include

► Excessive alcohol and caffeine (Both are diuretics that cause mineral loss.)

► Soft drinks (Their high phospate content promotes calcium loss.)

► Excessive protein in the diet

► Too much salt

► Refined sugar

► Smoking

MUSCULAR HEALTH

Muscle cells are subject to pre-programmed cell death just like those in the rest of the body (see page 19). However, muscles are still capable of growing in size and strength throughout life as long as they are exercised regularly. When muscles are not used enough, they tend to weaken and become smaller and dehydrated—a phenomenon called atrophy. Muscle cramps occur more frequently as you age, reflexes slow down, and if you are sedentary, many muscles become layered with fat. By age 65 or 70 the average body has doubled its fat content and halved its overall muscle mass. These changes can cause problems with the heart, circulation, and pelvic diaphragm, or floor—muscles that support the pelvic organs and prevent the bladder, uterus, and rectum from dropping downward. These muscles tend to relax and weaken during old age, resulting in various forms of prolapse.

ALTERNATIVE REMEDIES

A whole range of complementary therapies can help relieve aches, pains, and muscle and joint soreness. Many require a trained practitioner, but some, such as applying heat, you can do yourself:

► Heat is an age-old remedy for muscle soreness and general aching. Applying heat with a hot-water bottle or electric heating pad to a painful area or taking a warm bath can help relax you and relieve pain.

► Massage therapy is a tried-and-true method of relieving muscle soreness and stiffness.

► Yoga has long been used to strengthen, elongate, and realign muscles and bones. The gentle stretches and relaxing breathing techniques provide relief for many sufferers and can help prevent future problems. For more details about yoga, see page 116.

► Posture-based therapies, such as the Alexander technique (see page 116) or Pilates (see page 102), have a beneficial and preventive effect on diseases of the musculoskeletal system. Learning these techniques requires the help of a qualified instructor.

EXERCISE FOR MUSCULAR PROBLEMS

Much stiffness and muscular tension can be relieved with regular exercise. This does not have to involve expensive equipment or club memberships. Everyday activities can be tailored to your needs.

PROBLEM	EXERCISE
Grasping small objects, such as a door handle	Practice squeezing a small foam rubber ball to strengthen your fingers. An activity such as kneading dough may also help.
Getting up from a chair	Stiffness in the knees and lower back can be eased with stretching exercises, stepping up and down, and bending forward.
Carrying heavy objects	Build up your strength using small weights.
Walking up stairs	Bend and straighten your legs while sitting for any length of time.
Reaching up	Stretch your hands and arms down behind your back.
Twisting left or right	Reach backward at waist height to improve suppleness.

EXERCISE

Exercise is a major part of keeping bones, joints, and muscles healthy. Of particular benefit to the bones is weight-bearing exercise, like jogging, aerobics, dancing, tennis, and brisk walking, because it increases their density. Weight-bearing exercise also helps maintain good muscle function and limber joint movement

Non-weight-bearing exercise, such as swimming, will not strengthen the bones, but if you suffer from joint or back pain, swimming can be of great benefit. Because water supports your weight, there is no strain on the joints while you are exercising. Flexibility—the range of movement in a joint—is also improved by swimming and by simple stretching exercises. Doing some kind of stretching every day will increase elasticity in the surrounding muscles and tendons and tighten supporting ligaments.

Exercises that increase muscle mass are beneficial at any age. A study at Tufts University in Massachusetts analyzed the effects of a 12-week exercise program on muscle mass and strength. The results showed that it was possible to increase strength by 200 percent and muscle mass by 15 percent in men aged 60 to 70. A similar result was shown in women aged 87 to 96.

HORMONE THERAPY

Hormone replacement therapy (HRT) helps prevent osteoporosis (bone thinning) in postmenopausal women. However, it may increase the risk of breast cancer in some. For those who cannot take HRT, soy products like tofu, which contain a plant form of estrogen (isoflavones), may help prevent osteoporosis when combined with exercise. Calcitonin, a thyroid hormone that regulates calcium metabolism and inhibits the loss of calcium from bones, also halts osteoporosis. It may actually increase bone density.

BACKACHE

Backache is a common affliction, especially in older people. At least 80 percent of North Americans suffer an occasional backache, and for 15 percent the problem is chronic. The fact that humans stand upright places strain on the 33 vertebrae of the spine and the complex structure of muscles, cartilage, and tendons that holds them together, especially if posture is not perfect.

Most back pain occurs in the lower back because this area is the focus of much of the strain imposed by poor posture and lifting movements. Strain can be caused by an event that seems trivial at the time, like tripping over a carpet or bending over to pet the dog. Other back injuries have more obvious causes, such as picking up a heavy object in an improper way.

To relieve back pain, bed rest on a firm mattress with a pillow under your bent knees is often effective, as is applying ice to the painful area. A corset that constricts the movement of the back is good for short-term relief, but if used over a long period, it can make back muscles flabby and cause more pain in the long run.

Current advice is that people with back pain should begin gentle exercises to improve strength as soon as possible after an injury. The best way to prevent backache in the first place is to exercise regularly and maintain good posture (see below).

COPING WITH PAIN

If you suffer a sudden attack of back pain, lie down to take the pressure off your back, adopting any position that is comfortable but changing position frequently. Do not put more than two pillows under your head because the elevation may strain your neck and cause more discomfort.

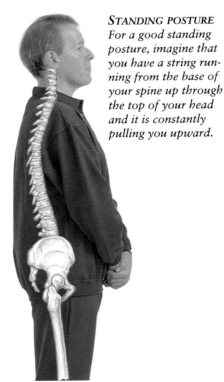

STANDING POSTURE
For a good standing posture, imagine that you have a string running from the base of your spine up through the top of your head and it is constantly pulling you upward.

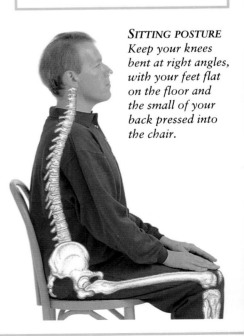

SITTING POSTURE
Keep your knees bent at right angles, with your feet flat on the floor and the small of your back pressed into the chair.

ARTHRITIS

Arthritis is a joint disease that can be extremely painful, even crippling. The word *arthritis,* which means "inflammation of a joint" is an umbrella term for more than 100 different conditions that affect joints and connective tissues throughout the body. The most common forms are osteoarthritis (OA) and rheumatoid arthritis (RA). Osteoarthritis is the result of joint cartilage deteriorating naturally with age and overuse. Rheumatoid arthritis is caused by the body's natural defenses—antibodies—attacking the connective tissue, making it swell up.

The role of diet in aggravating or improving arthritic conditions is still being studied, but many people have obtained relief by making changes in their eating habits or taking certain supplements (see box, far right). You can experiment to see what works for you. An elimination diet under the guidance of an allergist may turn up an allergy to one or more foods that is triggering RA, and elimination of the culprits should relieve symptoms.

Many naturopaths recommend that arthritis sufferers eat a whole-food diet high in vegetables and fruits and low in refined carbohydrates, meat, and saturated fat.

Some people find that cutting out dairy products reduces the extent of arthritic inflammation and pain, but care must be taken to maintain calcium intake from other sources.

Keeping weight under control is important. Excessive weight puts added strain on joints and will aggravate any kind of arthritis.

Putting all joints through range-of-motion exercises every day will help keep them mobile and functioning well. A physical therapist can help you devise a program. Swimming is a good exercise for arthritis sufferers because it does not put strain on the joints. The gentle exercises of yoga and t'ai chi are also recommended because they strengthen muscles around the joints and promote flexibility. When combined with meditation, they help reduce physical stress and manage pain as well.

As important as exercise is, it has to be balanced with rest because fatigue exacerbates arthritis. A cane helps relieve stress on hips and knees.

Hydrotherapy, including hot and cold wet packs, mineral baths, mud packs, and powerful directional showers, can improve circulation, help relieve stiffness, and possibly slow the deterioration of tissue.

Some studies have shown that an extract from the New Zealand green-lipped mussel appears to stop neutrophils from attacking healthy tissue in the joints of people with rheumatoid arthritis. The extract is a glycoprotein that blocks the action of neutrophils, white blood cells that trigger the immune system into action after injury or infection.

SUPPLEMENTS

The supplements below have helped many arthritis sufferers. Consult your doctor if you choose to try any of them. They could interfere with your medications; also advice is needed about dosage.

▶ Vitamins C, E, and niacin (in the form of niacinamide) are recommended for osteoarthritis.

▶ Zinc, copper, and vitamin B_6 are advised for rheumatoid arthritis.

▶ Omega-3 fatty acids in the form of fishoil or flaxseed oil capsules may help reduce inflammation.

▶ Gamma linoleic acid, contained in capsules of evening primrose oil, help reduce inflammation.

▶ Two sulfates, glucosamine and chondroitin, help renew cartilage and improve flexibility.

OSTEOARTHRITIS AND RHEUMATOID ARTHRITIS

Aromatherapists have a number of treatments they recommend for arthritis, depending upon which type you suffer from. All essential oils should be mixed with a carrier oil, like sesame or almond, before being applied to the skin. For a full-body massage, mix 20 to 25 drops of essential oil with 50 ml (about 2 fl oz) of the carrier oil.

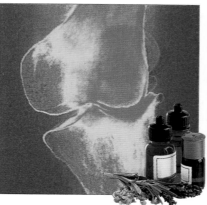

RHEUMATOID ARTHRITIS
For rheumatoid arthritis aromatherapists recommend massaging the affected joints with a carrier oil containing a couple of drops of rosemary, chamomile, camphor, juniper, or lavender oil.

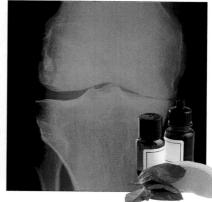

OSTEOARTHRITIS
For osteoarthritis aromatherapists advise mixing camphor and mint oils with sesame oil and using the mixture for a massage, or adding a couple of drops of lemon essential oil to your bath or to an oil burner.

Genitourinary System

The genitourinary system is a complex structure that performs some widely differing tasks. Keeping the system healthy is important for maintaining general health, as well as for avoiding discomfort and interruption of your sex life.

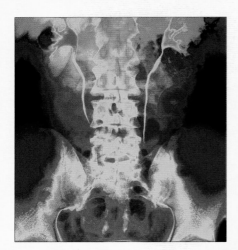

THE URINARY TRACT (UT)
The urinary tract is made up of the kidneys (top, in green), the bladder (bottom, in red and blue), and the ureters, which connect the kidneys and bladder.

GENITOURINARY HEALTH

The urinary system excretes waste as urea, which is diluted by water. Older people are not able to produce urine as dilute as that of younger people, and the resulting higher concentration of urea may cause discomfort. Older men are particularly vulnerable to disorders of the prostate, which often enlarges and puts pressure on the bladder. In fact, it is estimated that 90 percent of older men suffer some degree of prostate enlargement. Women become more vulnerable to genitourinary problems after menopause.

KEYS TO HEALTH

▶ As you grow older, you may have to pay more attention to your genitourinary system to prevent or deal with problems.

▶ Have regular checkups to catch any problems before they develop or become serious.

▶ To keep the system flushed out, drink at least eight glasses of water and other nonalcoholic beverages every day.

▶ Avoid excessive intake of alcohol and refined sugar.

URINARY PROBLEMS

The genitourinary system is made up of the kidneys, bladder, and genital organs. Each kidney is connected to the bladder by a tube called the ureter, which can become narrowed or blocked and cause serious problems if not treated. The bladder is normally very elastic, but with age it becomes more rigid. Coughing, sneezing, or pressure from the bowel may overcome the muscle's resistance and cause incontinence. Women are more prone to incontinence in later years when their pelvic muscles sag and the bladder shifts position. They are also more susceptable to urinary infections.

THE URINARY SYSTEM
The job of the urinary system is to filter excess water and salts out of the blood and store them until they can be released.

STONES
Stones, or calculi, may form in the kidney or bladder, obstructing the flow of urine and causing inflammation and pain. Stones can be removed surgically, but most are broken up with ultrasound.

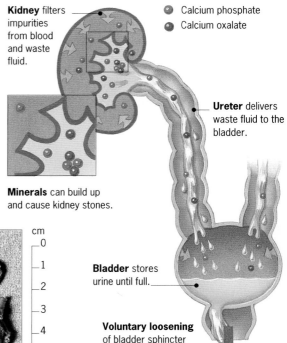

Kidney filters impurities from blood and waste fluid.

● Calcium phosphate
● Calcium oxalate

Ureter delivers waste fluid to the bladder.

Minerals can build up and cause kidney stones.

Bladder stores urine until full.

Voluntary loosening of bladder sphincter lets urine out.

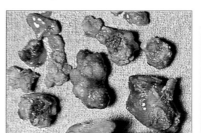

cm
0
1
2
3
4
5

MALE GENITOURINARY PROBLEMS

Men are particularly prone to stones forming in the bladder and the kidneys. To prevent kidney stones or avoid a recurrence of them, you should keep your system flushed out by drinking a lot of fluid—2 to 3 liters (quarts) of liquid a day. Some doctors advise even more. A dietary factor that may help is to cut back on such leafy greens as spinach, beet greens, and chard, as well as tea, chocolate, and many nuts, which are high in oxalate, a major component of many stones.

Enlargement of the male prostate gland affects almost all men over the age of 50 and can cause some problems. The prostate surrounds the upper part of the urethra (the pipe that leads from the bladder to the penis). When it enlarges, a man can have difficulty as he begins to urinate and may have a frequent need to urinate as well. The gland can also become infected, characterized by fever, lower back and groin pain, and frequent painful urination. Sometimes, too, the bladder does not empty completely after urinating, increasing the likelihood of bladder infections.

Symptoms of prostate enlargement can also be an indication of cancer. This is rare in younger men but fairly common in old age. Prostatectomy—removal of the prostate—is the most common operation performed on 60- to 70-year-old men. If you have any symptoms of prostate trouble, it is advisable to have a checkup.

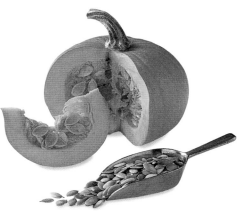

PROSTATE PROBLEMS

The following can help relieve some prostate problems:

▶ An infusion of buchu leaves, which have anti-inflammatory properties, can relieve inflammation of the prostate or bladder.

▶ An extract of saw palmetto can reduce some of the symptoms of prostate enlargement. However, it should be taken only under the guidance of a physician, because it may interfere with prescription drugs for prostate problems.

▶ Eating soybeans and soy products and foods high in zinc, such as seafood, meat, and fortified cereals, may help diminish the symptoms of an enlarged prostate.

PUMPKIN SEEDS
A daily intake of pumpkin seeds is believed to help prevent prostate disorders or relieve some of the symptoms. This effect may be due in part to their high content of certain amino acids that have been shown to affect symptoms.

SEXUAL HEALTH IN MEN

Healthy elderly men, unlike elderly women, remain physically capable of reproduction. In 1995, for instance, Englishman Bill Lampard became a father at the age of 93. Unfortunately, he died when his daughter was only five months old—leaving a widow 53 years younger.

Men continue to have erections all their lives, although in later years the erections may be less rigid and less frequent than those of younger men. There is no reason, however, why anyone should not enjoy fulfilling sex throughout life.

Impotence is a problem that affects approximately 10 percent of the male population, though almost every man will experience it at some time. The condition is not necessarily age related but can be caused by various factors, such as stress, diabetes, alcohol, or heart problems. If you experience impotence over a period longer than two weeks, you should see a doctor; it may be due to a physical problem that can be effectively treated.

In addition to regular exercise and a healthy diet that is low in saturated fat, there are several measures you can take to prevent or combat impotence. First of all, if you smoke, give it up. Try to maintain a consistent, healthy weight and cut down your alcohol intake. Find out if any of your prescriptions could be causing problems; impotence is a common side effect of certain drugs. Also, try to address any emotional difficulties you may be experiencing; stress is a common cause of impotence, and relieving tension can be an effective cure.

MALE MENOPAUSE

During menopause in women there is a decline in certain hormones. Male hormone levels also decrease with age, but in a far more gradual manner than those of women. Some doctors are convinced, however, that the decline is enough to cause a "male menopause" with symptoms such as irritability, lack of sexual desire and ability, and depression. Many of these same doctors also believe that men can benefit from the male hormone testosterone, administered in the form of a patch or injection. This treatment is controversial, however, because there are indications that increased testosterone levels may be a causative factor in testicular cancer.

VAGINAL AND URINARY PROBLEMS

A reduction in the level of estrogen that occurs at menopause (see below) makes the female genitourinary system increasingly vulnerable to attack from infectious organisms. The main threats are yeasts, such as *Candida albicans*, and bacteria, mainly *E. coli*, which can be transferred from the rectum.

Yeast overgrowths cause candidiasis, which occurs when the delicate balance of normal vaginal flora is upset. There may be a thick white discharge accompanied by itchiness and pain on urination or sexual intercourse. One natural cure for candidiasis is yogurt with live cultures. If you are suffering, eat one cup daily and try dipping a tampon in plain live yogurt and leaving it in the vagina for an hour—no more.

Bacterial infections are also common—cystitis in the urinary tract and bacterial vaginosis (BV) in the vagina.

Cystitis sufferers should drink lots of fluid and try to make their urine alkaline by taking a citrate of calcium, potassium, or sodium (with the advice of a doctor) three or four times a day. Drinking cranberry or blueberry juice is also beneficial because both prevent bacteria from adhering to the bladder walls.

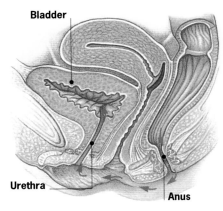

Bladder

Urethra

Anus

◀— **Pathway of infection**

ALTERNATIVE REMEDIES

There are many alternative remedies for vaginal and urinary problems. Herbal medicine in particular has a vast body of lore regarding such disorders.

► For general urinary relief, wintergreen, blackberry root, or coleus is beneficial.

► Goldenseal is used for its anti-infective properties.

► Uva ursi is recommended to improve urine flow.

► For cystitis an infusion of buchu or parsley leaves is advised.

► Tea tree oil and calendula pessaries relieve candidiasis.

PATH OF INFECTION
The proximity of the vagina, urethra, and anus means that gut bacteria like E. coli *do not have far to travel to infect the genitourinary system.*

MENOPAUSE

Probably the major event for older women in terms of their reproductive health is menopause. This signals the end of fertility for a woman. The ovaries stop releasing ova (egg cells) and cease to produce hormones at their previously high levels. Women's levels of the hormone estrogen do not drop to zero after menopause, but they do fall to about the same level as in men of the same age. In Western countries menopause used to be treated as an illness. This is far from the case now, and it is more accurately seen as a natural part of normal human development.

The most obvious sign of menopause is the ceasing of menstrual periods. This may happen gradually over time, with periods becoming more and more irregular, and some symptoms of menopause may appear. This transition period is known as perimenopause.

Common symptoms associated with menopause are hot flashes, drying of the vagina, night sweats, poor memory, difficulty with concentration, osteoporosis, depression, anxiety, irritability, loss of libido, tension, insomnia, headaches, dry skin, dry hair, weight gain, tiredness, palpitations, and aching limbs and joints. It is rare for a menopausal woman to suffer all of the indications, however, and most symptoms will diminish or disappear over time.

DID YOU KNOW?
China claims to have no cases of menopausal depression or other psychiatric disturbance associated with menopause. One possible explanation advanced by anthropologists is that this is because menopause signifies the entrance into a higher status in the culture for Chinese women.

NATURAL THERAPIES

Some natural products have been shown to reduce common symptoms of menopause. These are especially beneficial to women who cannot take hormone replacement therapy. They include

► Black cohosh capsules or extract

► Ginseng capsules or extract

► Evening primrose or black currant oil to help prevent bloating

► Soy products or capsules of their isoflavones

► Red raspberry, damiana, licorice, or valerian tea

► Vitamins (see opposite page)

Limiting or abstaining from nicotine, alcohol, and caffeine will help mitigate hot flashes. Getting regular exercise will lift mood, strengthen bones, help prevent weight gain, and lower the risk of heart disease.

VITAMINS THAT MAY BENEFIT MENOPAUSAL PROBLEMS

VITAMIN	SOURCES	PROBLEMS
Vitamin A (Retinol and carotene)	Liver, salmon, egg yolks, broccoli, carrrots, leafy greens, sweet potatoes, apricots, cantaloupes	Excessive menstrual bleeding, cervical abnormalities, fibrocystic disease, cancer of the breast, leukoplakia and other skin conditions
Folic Acid (Vitamin B complex)	Liver, yeast, leafy greens, legumes, broccoli and other crucifers, avocados	Cervical abnormalities and cancer, osteoporosis, diabetes mellitus
Vitamin B_3 (Niacin)	Meat, poultry, seafood, eggs, legumes, milk, whole-grain breads and cereals	Hyperlipidemia (high concentration of blood fat), hypoglycemia (low blood sugar)
Vitamin B_6 (Pyridoxine)	Meat, poultry, fish, leafy greens, whole-grain cereals, soybeans	Deficiency as a result of taking HRT, cervical abnormalities and cancer, diabetes mellitus
Vitamin B_{12} (Cyanocobalamin)	Meat, poultry, fish, eggs, milk, B_{12}-enriched soy products (no plants contain B_{12})	Anxiety, depression, mood swings, fatigue
Vitamin C (Ascorbic acid)	Citrus fruits, kiwis, berries, melons, broccoli, green peppers, potatoes	Excessive menstrual bleeding, cervical abnormalities and cancer, chloasma
Vitamin D (Calciferol)	Oily fish and fish liver oils; egg yolks; fortified milk, margarine, and butter; exposure to sunlight	Poor calcium absorption, leading to an increase in the risk of osteoporosis
Vitamin E (Tocopherol)	Vegetable oils, leafy greens, nuts, seeds, eggs, whole grains, fortified cereals and breads	Hot flashes, anxiety, vaginal problems (e.g., dryness), hypothyroidism, chloasma and other skin conditions, atherosclerosis, osteoarthritis, fibrocystic disease of the breast

POSTMENOPAUSAL PROBLEMS

Cells in the female genitourinary system have many receptors for estrogen. Before menopause, estrogen binds with them, stimulating cells and keeping the whole system strong and active. Lower levels of estrogen after menopause have several consequences.

Atrophy of the pelvic muscles is one consequence of low estrogen levels. This increases the risk of uterine prolapse because the uterus is no longer held so tightly in place. Genital atrophy—thinness and dryness of the vaginal membranes—also occurs, causing discomfort during sex, and it can lead to infection and vaginismus (painful vaginal contraction). Low estrogen levels also weaken the bladder sphincter, increasing the chances of incontinence, particularly under conditions in which pressure is exerted on the bladder—for instance, during coughing, sneezing, or laughing.

Another major postmenopausal problem is osteoporosis, or thinning of the bones (see pages 62–63).

CELL RECEPTORS
Estrogen receptors are found in cells of the genitourinary tract. When there is a plentiful supply of estrogen, it binds with the cells and keeps the system healthy and resistant to infections.

KEGEL EXERCISES

Women can control continence by strengthening the muscles of the pelvic floor, using exercises named after the doctor who first described them. These are often taught for the first time after pregnancy but are very useful in later life too. The idea is to contract the muscles that you use to stop passing urine. Doing this exercise many times a day will gradually strengthen your pelvic-floor muscles.

Cell membrane / Cell nucleus / Cell receptors / Estrogen

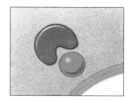

BEFORE MENOPAUSE *Estrogen molecules easily bind with the receptors in the cells.*

AFTER MENOPAUSE *The receptors cannot bind with estrogen, and the system becomes vulnerable.*

The Senses

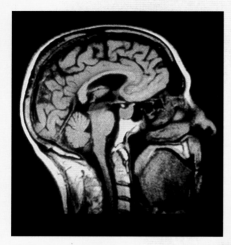

Your sense of smell
When your nose detects a smell, signals are sent to your brain, where they are processed to allow you to recognize and react to the smell.

THE EFFECTS OF AGING

All the senses deteriorate gradually during the aging process. It is estimated that one-third of people over the age of 65 in the Western world suffer presbycusis, or age-related hearing loss. Color perception also diminishes with age; an 80-year-old person needs about eight times as much light as a young one to see well. However, there are things you can do to minimize deterioration and to cope with a sense that is diminishing.

KEYS TO HEALTH

▶ Good nutrition is central to maintenance of your sensory equipment. Make sure that you get enough B vitamins, and vitamins A, C, D, and E. Consider supplements if your diet is inadequate, but consult a doctor first.

▶ Protect your hearing by wearing ear plugs in the vicinity of loud noises, such as street drilling and a hair dryer.

▶ Get regular checkups of your eyes and ears.

Keeping the five senses sharp is a concern for many people as they age. Your sight, hearing, smell, taste, and touch are all integral to a good quality of life. It is possible with certain care to minimize any deterioration that may occur.

HEARING

Hearing loss is generally thought to be the result of natural deterioration combined with lifelong exposure to environmental noise. Disease, drugs that affect hearing, and trauma may also contribute. The three delicate bones of the inner ear may become arthritic, or the sensitive hairs in the inner ear that pick up sound waves may degenerate. Another hearing problem is tinnitus, a condition in which a persistent ringing or buzzing noise is heard in the head or ears. This may be caused by disease, but in the majority of cases the cause is never found. Treatment for tinnitus includes hearing aids to increase other noise and mask the tinnitus and taking ginkgo biloba.

Deafness often develops gradually, so much so that a person's family often notices the hearing loss first. If you feel that your hearing is deteriorating or family members are constantly having to repeat things

EAR INFECTION

Earache can easily be treated with home remedies. If the pain is persistent, however (lasting more than two days), it is important to see a doctor.

▶ Always treat both ears if you have an infection.

▶ An ice pack will bring relief; press it against the affected ear.

▶ A hot-salt bag is a traditional remedy for earache: heat one cupful of salt in a warm oven for 15 minutes, place it in a cloth bag, and hold the bag against the ear for 30 minutes. A hot-water bottle, heating pad, or bag of oat hulls heated in a microwave also works.

to you, see your doctor to have your hearing checked. This will help rule out any other problems related to the ears, and treatment can be initiated if hearing loss has occurred.

HEARING AIDS

If you suffer from any degree of deafness, a hearing aid can help. Many are very small and unobtrusive and can be programmed for specific hearing problems. A hearing aid consists of a small microphone to pick up sounds and convert them to electric current, an amplifier to increase their strength, and a minute speaker to transmit sounds to the inner ear.

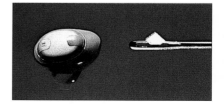

Miniature miracles
Hearing aids are now available that are so small they fit on a pinhead and are practically invisible.

SIGHT

The most obvious age-related change to eyes is a lessening of the elasticity of the internal lenses. As the lens hardens, focusing on close objects becomes more difficult—a condition called presbyopia. Holding a book about 7 cm (3 inches) from the eyes works fine for a young child; at the age of 40 the book may have to be held about 30 cm (12 inches) away, and at 60 it may have to be held at arm's length. This is why most older people require reading glasses. If reading small print is becoming less easy for you, have your eyes checked to determine the strength of reading lens needed.

As you age, the lens of your eye begins to yellow. This makes it more difficult to distinguish between light and dark shades of color, especially cool colors like green, blue, and violet because they are filtered out by the yellowing lens. Older eyes also take longer to adjust from a light to a dark environment, and as a result, older people see less well in the dark. You should take this into account, especially in regard to night driving.

Bright sunlight and ultraviolet light can produce a haze, or fluorescence, over aging eyes, so there is a greater need for older people to shade the eyes with hats. Regular eye examinations are essential as you grow older, not only to ensure you have the correct prescription for glasses, but also to check that you are free from more serious problems, such as glaucoma, cataracts, or corneal infections. All these conditions are treatable if caught early but can lead to blindness if allowed to develop.

Good diet is essential for maintaining normal vision. Vitamin A is an important component of retinal pigments, and an inadequate intake can result in night blindness. There is also evidence that eating vegetables rich in pigments called carotenoids can prevent degeneration of the macula, the area of the retina that is responsible for sharp, detailed vision.

POOR SIGHT

A few simple alterations to your home can make living with failing eyesight much easier.

▶ Fit more powerful lightbulbs in your light fixtures, especially reading lamps. If you suffer from glaucoma, however, use caution because strong lights can cause glare and dark shadows that may aggravate the condition.

▶ Never leave the house completely dark at night. Put night lights in the hallway and bathroom so if you need to get up in the night, you can see clearly.

▶ Stick fluorescent tape around light switches, plugs, door handles, and keyholes. This will make them more visible, especially in poor light.

▶ Explain any visual loss to your family and friends so they can help you make adjustments in your lifestyle.

BATES EYE METHOD

Dr. William H. Bates (1860–1931) was an ophthalmologist who developed a method of eyesight "training" with four basic exercises. Initially its purpose was to rest the eyes and prevent eyestrain, but he discovered that his techniques also helped people improve their sight. Before trying the exercises, remove glasses or contact lenses. Palming (see far right) rests the eyes; splashing (see right) stimulates circulation and reinvigorates eyes. Focusing improves focus; to practice it, hold one pencil near your eyes and one at arm's length and switch focus between them. Swinging helps relax the eye muscles. It is done by simply swaying your body and moving your eyes with it.

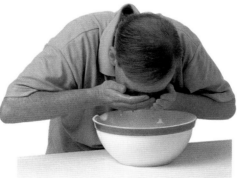

SPLASHING
First thing every morning, splash your closed eyes 20 times with warm water, then repeat with cold water. This will stimulate circulation. Just before going to bed, reverse this process, splashing your eyes 20 times with cold water and then 20 times with warm water.

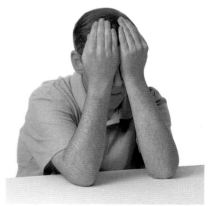

PALMING
Sit comfortably at a desk or table. Rest your elbows on the table and cover your closed eyes with your cupped palms. Picture in your mind a scene or object in great detail. Stay like this for about 10 minutes. Repeat twice a day or whenever your eyes feel tired.

TASTE AND SMELL

The senses of taste and smell are related; if one is damaged, the other will be compromised. Many older people begin to lose some ability in taste or smell or both from around the age of 60.

Your nose is divided into two parts: the external portion, which consists of bone and cartilage, and the inner chamber, where smells are detected and sent to the brain. Odor molecules pass up the nostrils with inflowing air, which is warmed as it passes over nasal bones called turbinates. The scent molecules are detected in an area called the olfactory epithelium, which is covered with mucus containing hairlike cilia. These cilia pick up odors entering the mucus layer, analyze them, and send the information to the brain.

Studies have shown that older people have a reduced ability to identify many smells, including some strong ones like coffee and menthol. This loss of smell is caused by age-related changes in the sensory cells that line the inner part of the nose.

The nerves that connect these cells with the brain may also degenerate.

People can identify hundreds of different flavors, but a large proportion of this range is dependent on the sense of smell working with the tastebuds. There are only four pure tastes: sweet, sour, bitter, and salty.

Taste is detected by the taste buds, which are in the papillae of the tongue's surface and on the roof of the mouth. Each taste bud is made up of clusters of cells that enclose a short, stiff taste hair. This hair protrudes into a taste pore close to the surface of the taste bud, which in turn relays information to the brain, where the taste is analyzed.

Studies have been conflicting about whether the number of taste buds on the tongue decreases with age. Some researchers believe that they decrease by as much as 80 percent. One thing they agree upon, however, is that one very important cause of deterioration in both taste and smell is the use of medications (see box, above). The main problem associated with loss of taste and smell is a decreased

enjoyment of food, which can affect the quality of life. More serious problems occur if diminished taste leads to dietary and nutritional deficiencies. An elderly person who is debilitated may find it difficult to regain weight that has been lost. Recent studies have even suggested that elderly people given flavor-enhanced food show improvement in their immune systems. Using more herbs and spices rather than salt is a healthy way to increase the flavor of food (see page 93).

TASTE DEPLETERS

More than 250 medications have been found to alter taste and smell in some way. These include large classes of drugs that are commonly prescribed for elderly people:

► Antihypertensives
► Antiasthmatics
► Sleeping medications
► Antibiotics
► Drugs used for diabetes, heart conditions, and Parkinson's disease

EATING WITH DIMINISHED TASTE AND SMELL

The ability to taste salty and bitter foods diminishes with age much more than with sweet foods, although older people who are not on any medication should have only a modest decrease in taste sensitivity. If you find yourself adding extra salt to food in order to taste it, reduced taste sensitivity might be the reason. It is not a good idea to eat too much salt; adding flavor with herbs and spices is better. In addition to the suggestions given below, try fresh ginger and lemon juice as flavor enhancers.

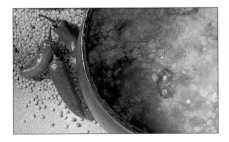

CHILIES
Chilies are used in Mexican and Asian cuisines. Their hot taste is thought to release endorphins—natural opiates that give a pleasurable sensation.

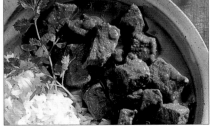

CURRIES
Asian cuisine incorporates a huge variety of spices, ranging from subtle to hot. These include cumin, coriander, and in Thai cooking, lemon grass.

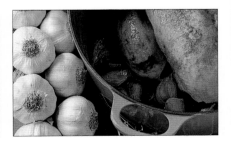

GARLIC
An essential component of many European dishes, garlic is both flavorful and renowned for its health-giving properties. Use it as often as possible.

TOUCH

With a surface area of about 1.7 square meters (6 square feet) for an average adult, the skin is the largest sensory organ in the body. There are different types of skin on different parts of the body, and they contain various densities of skin receptors that transmit the sensations of vibration, temperature, touch, and pressure to the brain.

The sensitivity of skin decreases as you grow older, so that you become less able to identify different sensations by touch. Your threshold for pain and temperature also increases—that is, you are able to tolerate higher temperatures and greater levels of pain than before. This can be dangerous because you are more likely to suffer some form of injury if you do not register pain or cannot feel extreme temperatures.

Touch is the first of our senses to develop in the womb, and our need for it continues throughout life. Older people who live alone often go for days without being touched. Studies have shown that those who are touched regularly—whether the touching is done by a friend, a relative, a nurse, or other caregiver—take less time to recover from illness. Massage is an excellent therapy for older people. Not only does it fulfill the need for touch but it also improves circulation, relieves pain, and can improve the mobility and flexibility of the body.

TACTILE THERAPY

The importance of touching and being touched is often under-rated, not just as a therapeutic tool but as part of everyday life. For older people who may have lost some acuity in their other senses, such as hearing and vision, touch—even a casual hug—can be a rewarding substitute.

Simple measures, such as caressing a pet, can make a big difference to both mental and physical health. Studies confirm that elderly pet owners, particularly those who live alone, have relatively less depression and a lower incidence of illness than those who do not have a pet.

MASSAGE TO HEIGHTEN SENSITIVITY

An excellent way to reduce stress and stimulate your senses is for you and your partner to massage each other. Set aside at least an hour for a massage session in a warm, quiet, private room. Use warm massage oil, perhaps with a few drops of aromatherapy oil added, and apply it with firm, even strokes.

Massage is generally made up of three types of stroke. Effleurage, or long sweeping movements; tapotement, or chopping movements applied with the sides of the hands; and petrissage, largely kneading movements. Aspects of two of the three techniques are shown below left.

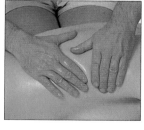

KNEADING
Firm rolling of the flesh between the hands breaks down muscle tension.

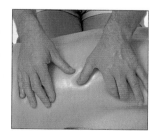

CUPPING
Firm, not hard, slapping with cupped hands increases blood supply to the muscles.

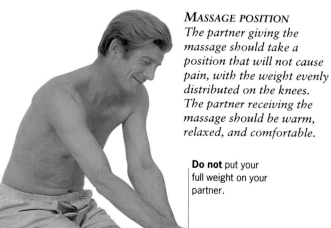

MASSAGE POSITION
The partner giving the massage should take a position that will not cause pain, with the weight evenly distributed on the knees. The partner receiving the massage should be warm, relaxed, and comfortable.

Do not put your full weight on your partner.

Illnesses of the Whole body

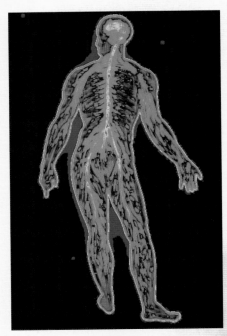

THE NERVOUS SYSTEM
The brain and spinal cord branch into the peripheral nervous system that runs throughout your body.

THE EFFECTS OF AGING
The human body becomes less resistant to illness and injury as it ages. A reduction in the level of hormones, the weakening of the immune system, cellular damage, and a buildup of toxins over time all take their toll on health. In later life hereditary problems or old injuries may also show their effects for the first time.

KEYS TO HEALTH
▶ Try to avoid the major carcinogens of modern life—mainly smoking but also overexposure to the sun, air pollutants, and other substances that are known to be carcinogenic.

▶ Eat foods every day that are high in antioxidants (see page 86).

▶ Learn how to check for and recognize early signs of cancer.

As you grow older, you become more susceptible to conditions that affect the whole body—not just particular systems. Among them are cancer, diabetes, and problems with the nervous system or regulation of body temperature.

CANCER

Cancer is an abnormal growth of cells that produces malignant masses, or tumors, that can spread around the body. The condition can quickly become lifethreatening if diseased cells invade any vital tissue, such as a large blood vessel or major organ. The course of cancer depends on where it originates and where it spreads to. Regular screening to catch cancer in its early stages can lower the risk of its overwhelming the body. The incidence of the disease rises rapidly with age, but it is reassuring to note that age does not affect responses to treatment.

Although cancer is usually treated with surgery, radiation therapy, and/or chemotherapy, alternative approaches can play a vital role alongside conventional treatment, both for relieving pain and for bolstering defenses in the battle against the disease.

Many patients who have beaten cancer advocate the therapy known as creative visualization, in which white blood cells are pictured doing battle with invasive carcinogens and cancerous cells—and winning. There are quite a few documented cases of people who have helped themselves cope with their illness through visualization.

The antioxidant vitamins, A, C, and E, as well as selenium and zinc (see page 86), are believed to have a preventive effect against cancer because they eradicate the free radicals that can damage cells and strengthen the immune system.

Eating plenty of fruits and vegetables that contain these nutrients could be the most important anticancer measure you take during your life.

Smoking is the main cause of lung cancer, now one of the most common diseases in the Western world. Smoking also causes other health problems, including lowering the effectiveness of the immune system, damaging the heart, and accelerating the aging of skin. There are many approaches to quitting smoking, ranging from nicotine patches to acupuncture to hypnotherapy. Whatever you choose, it is best to try to avoid situations in which you know you will want to smoke.

PREVENTION IS BETTER THAN CURE

In the case of cancer, screening and early detection are very important. Early diagnosis and treatment may save your life. There are some self tests that you should perform regularly to reassure yourself that you are disease-free or to detect early treatable signs of disease. Other screenings should be done by a medical practitioner on a regular basis. Most of these tests cause a minimum of discomfort and are becoming more accurate all the time. After age 65, people should have cancer screening every two years.

Breast cancer screening
Particularly after the age of 50, women should have a mammogram of their breasts annually. It can be done at a local hospital, a doctor's office, or a special screening unit. In addition to this annual checkup, you should examine your own breasts every month. Lie down and feel for any lumps or changes in the breast tissue. Look closely at your breasts to see if there are any changes. If you notice anything different, see a doctor for a further checkup.

BREAST EXAMINATION
Be alert for unusual swellings in breast tissue or darkening or inverting of your nipples.

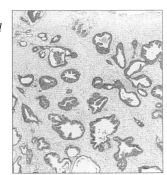

Cervical cancer screening
A regular Pap smear is important for detecting early signs of cervical cancer, which most commonly develops between ages 40 and 55. For the test a sample of cells is gathered from the cervix and sent to a laboratory for analysis. Women should have this test every two to three years, more often if they are at high risk. If abnormal cells are discovered, they can be removed by laser treatment, freezing, or hot cauterization.

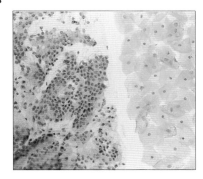

CERVICAL SMEAR
Despite differences in shape and color, all the cells in the above image are healthy and cancer free.

Prostate cancer screening
Cancer of the prostate gland, which surrounds the neck of the bladder and urethra (see page 67), is one of the most common male cancers. You should have your prostate checked regularly by a doctor, especially if you experience any change in urinary habits, and have a prostate specific antigen (PSA) test annually. As with many cancers, prostate cancer can be effectively treated if caught early enough.

PROSTATE CELLS
The white, irregularly shaped areas in this image are cancerous cells, which are surrounded by healthy cells, shown in red.

Testicular cancer screening
Men should check their testicles regularly for early signs of testicular cancer. Although the disease is more common among younger men, it is by no means exclusive to them. Testicular cancer can be successfully treated if caught early enough—the cure rate is 95 to 100 percent. By acting quickly, you have a good chance of saving your life.

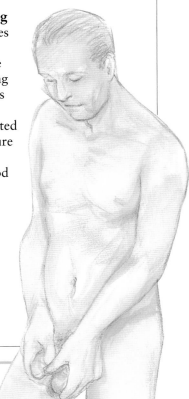

SELF TESTING
To check yourself, carefully feel the entire surface of each testicle at least once a month. Any lump should be checked by a doctor.

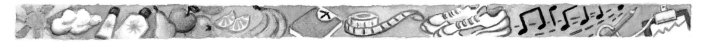

ARE YOU AT RISK FOR CANCER?

Although a general cure for cancer has yet to be found, medical science is now very knowledgeable about the causes of many forms of the disease. Knowing if you are in a high risk group and changing some of your habits accordingly may help you prevent cancer. There are various lifestyle changes that you can make.

LIFESTYLE FACTOR	POSSIBLE EFFECT	ACTION
Have you already had cancer?	Any cancerous cell division can spread to other parts of the body; this is called metastasis.	Having suffered cancer, you should have frequent checkups to ensure that the cancer has not affected other parts of your body.
Are you over 50 years old?	As the body ages, cells accumulate mutations and do not function as effectively; the immune system becomes weaker.	Regular checkups and a healthy diet and lifestyle can reduce risks.
Do you smoke?	The tar and other ingredients in cigarettes have a carcinogenic effect on the lungs, throat, and mouth. Low-tar cigarettes are now considered to be just as dangerous as high-tar brands.	It is vital to stop smoking as soon as possible. This will bring about immediate improvements. Passive smokers are also at risk and should avoid smoky atmospheres.
Do you drink to excess?	A high intake of alcohol has been linked to many cancers, including cancer of the liver, gall bladder, and mouth.	Although alcohol in moderation can be good for you, you should not exceed the guidelines for safe alcohol limits (see page 91).
Is your diet healthy?	Smoke and charring from grilled foods can be carcinogenic. Mold on food may also cause cancer. Peanut mold contains aflatoxin, one of the most potent carcinogens known.	Eat charcoal-grilled food only occasionally. Avoid moldy foods, especially moldy peanuts. Increase your intake of fruits and vegetables for their antioxidant content. Limit your intake of fatty and sugary foods in order to maintain a healthy weight.
Are you overweight?	The more excess weight you carry, the greater your risk of developing cancer. It is not known if this is due to the excess weight itself or perhaps to poor diet or later detection.	Maintain a healthy weight with regular exercise and a healthy diet. Do not lose too much weight, however; being underweight also increases the risk of some cancers.
Are you often exposed to the sun?	Skin becomes weaker and slightly thinner as it ages and is more vulnerable to the effects of damaging ultraviolet light. Depletion of the world's ozone layer has added to the problem of skin cancer, as has the increase in vacations taken in sunny places by people from colder climates, whose skins are not used to and thus are more vulnerable to the sun.	Always wear sunscreen and a hat when you are outdoors in the sun. Never let yourself get sunburned, and if you are regularly in the sun, check for newly developed moles and moles that have changed shape or color or have become sore or itchy. Avoid prolonged exposure to the sun.
Are you highly stressed?	Parallels have been drawn between those who lead frenetic and highly stressed lifestyles and the incidence of cancer. Your state of mind can promote physical changes, such as in the immune response, muscular tension, heart rate, and the output of various hormones.	Take up a stress-relieving activity, such as meditation, yoga, or t'ai chi, to improve your peace of mind and strengthen your immunity.
Are you at risk from the environment?	Air pollution has been found to add to the risks of cancer. People living and working in industrial areas may be at risk from carcinogenic chemicals.	Wear protective clothing in the workplace and limit exposure to chemicals. Always follow safety guidelines carefully and thoroughly.
For women only: Did menopause begin after 50?	The later the onset of menopause, the greater the risk of certain cancers.	Women who have a late onset of menopause should have regular cancer checkups.
Have any close family members had cancer?	Genetic susceptibility to cancer has been well documented.	Research the medical history of your family and have regular checkups.

DIABETES

Diabetes occurs when the hormone insulin fails to adequately play its role in the body. There are different forms. With the insulin-dependent type, little or no insulin is produced by the body and insulin injections are necessary. A more common form is adult-onset diabetes, which develops primarily in people over 40 and can shorten life by as much as 30 percent if left untreated. In adult-onset diabetes, insulin production does not cease entirely, but the body fails to utilize it properly. Insulin injections are not usually required, and the condition is controlled through diet and sometimes medication. Insulin plays a vital role in the

body (see diagram below). Glucose imbalance caused by lack of insulin action can result in deterioration of many of the body's organs and tissues. Diabetics are especially prone to problems of the kidneys, eyes, and circulation. Diabetics are also more likely to develop such difficulties as heart disease earlier than average.

Evidence suggests that adult-onset diabetes can be prevented by eating few refined carbohydrates, getting adequate fiber, maintaining a healthy weight, and keeping fit with regular exercise. Some 9 out of 10 adults who develop diabetes are overweight or obese. (See page 89 for more information on diabetes.)

DIABETES
The healthy working of the body depends on maintaining a delicate balance of blood sugar levels. In diabetes this balance is upset by a deficiency of insulin or inefficiency in the way it functions.

⬡ Carbohydrates
▭ Glucose
● Insulin

Stomach juices break down carbohydrates in food.

Complex carbohydrates are converted to simple sugars.

Insulin normally promotes absorption of glucose by the liver and muscles.

Diabetes symptoms: excessive urination, constant thirst and hunger, unexplained weight loss, fatigue, accelerated degeneration of small blood vessels, disordered lipid metabolism

Food is eaten.

Pancreas fails to supply enough insulin to cope with the amount of glucose.

Lack of insulin leaves unstored glucose in the bloodstream, leading to high blood sugar.

DEGENERATIVE PROBLEMS

Degenerative disorders of the brain and nervous system, like Parkinson's disease, multiple sclerosis, and Alzheimer's disease, can strike younger people but are more prevalent in those who are older. They can be debilitating and dramatically alter the quality of life. Parkinson's is characterized by a rhythmic tremor, progressive muscle stiffening, and an unstable gait. Multiple sclerosis can have some of the same symptoms, plus memory, vision, and hearing loss.

Although knowledge of what causes these problems and treatments for them are in their infancy,

it is thought that B-group vitamins play a vital role in the maintenance of the brain and nervous system. The antioixidant vitamins C and E, omega-3 fatty acids, and gingko biloba may also be beneficial in slowing the onset or progression of Alzheimer's and Parkinson's.

Motor neuron illnesses make the body less flexible and cause muscles to atrophy and weaken. The meditation, stretching, and balancing aspects of yoga and t'ai chi can help people keep their muscles toned and supple and encourage relaxation, which can calm symptoms.

EPILEPSY

Epilepsy is caused by irregular and chaotic electrical activity in the brain. It is estimated that 4 out of 1,000 people develop epilepsy later in life, perhaps as a result of a brain injury, an infection, or a tumor.

There are several types, but the two most common ones are grand mal and petit mal. The seizure that characterizes grand mal epilepsy can be very frightening. The person falls to the floor and then has a brief period of violent twitching and jerking that affects the whole body. You should not try to restrain a person during a seizure (see box, right).

Petit mal seizures are characterized by staring and momentary loss of awareness, which may appear to be daydreaming. These last only a few seconds and occur mainly in children, who often outgrow them. It is best to ignore such seizures.

For at least two-thirds of epileptics there is no known cause or identifiable brain abnormality, though stress may trigger an attack in some people. Epilepsy cannot be cured, but it can be controlled with anticonvulsant drugs. A special ketogenic (very low-carbohydrate) diet may be proposed for anyone who does not respond to medication. Healthy eating, adequate rest, and relaxation are advised to maintain good health and minimize stress. For safety, sufferers should wear a tag that identifies them as epileptic.

FIRST AID FOR SEIZURES

Do not restrain someone who is having a seizure unless the movements are dangerous to the person or others. Contrary to popular advice, you should not try to place anything in the person's mouth. This will not prevent biting of the tongue, as once was supposed, but could cause the tongue to block the airway.

After a seizure the muscles relax, which may lead to a loss of bladder and bowel control. A sufferer often sleeps afterward and should be left to do so, as long as he or she is safe and comfortable. Check now and then to see that everything is all right.

HYPOTHERMIA

Hypothermia is a life-threatening drop in the body's temperature to below 35°C (95°F), which occurs when the body loses heat faster than it can generate it. The condition most often results from exposure to frigid water or weather (alcohol and inadequate attire in particular can be a fatal combintion in subzero weather), but many cases occur indoors in temperatures ranging from 10° to 16°C (50° to 60°F). Older people are especially vulnerable because of poor circulation, decreased sensitivity to cold, and lessened ability to shiver.

If someone you know shows signs of hypothermia, call for an ambulance or take the person to an emergency facility. In the meantime, take first-aid measures (see box, right).

To prevent hypothermia, older people should wear layers of clothing, even indoors, during cold weather and keep the thermostat at a minimum of 20°C (68°F) during the day. If room temperature drops to 14°C (57°F) or lower at night, it's a good idea to wear socks and gloves, as well as layers of clothing, to bed.

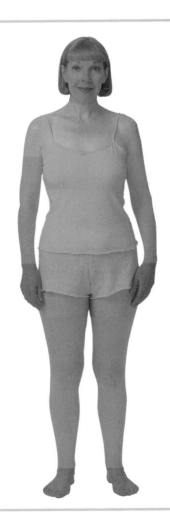

TELLTALE SIGNS

Signs of hypothermia include blue finger and toe nails, blue lips, uncoordinated movements, slurred speech, confused responses, slow breathing, and a weak pulse. The sufferer may seem inattentive and want only to sleep.

He or she may complain of cold extremities, but you should not rub the skin because this may damage tissues that are not protected by normal blood circulation. Help the person to warm up slowly by wrapping him or her in a blanket and raising the temperature in the room. If the patient is conscious, offer warm tea or soup but nothing alcoholic.

HOW THE BODY COOLS
The cooling process begins with the extremities—the hands and feet—and gradually extends to the trunk as the circulatory system protects the heart by drawing the resources of warm blood back to the torso. An indication of dangerous hypothermia is when areas that are usually warm, such as the abdomen or the insides of the thighs, feel cold to the touch.

CHAPTER 4

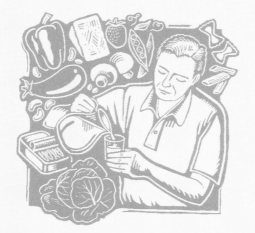

YOU ARE WHAT YOU EAT

If you eat too much junk food or don't eat enough of the foods that contain nutrients needed for the optimum functioning of your body, you become vulnerable to ill health and disease, particularly as you grow older. A well-balanced diet is essential for maintaining a body that can run trouble-free well into old age.

A HEALTHY DIET

As you grow older, it becomes more important than ever for your diet to be healthy and balanced. The foods you choose should be rich in the nutrients that protect you against disease.

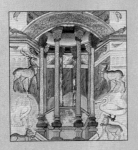
Advancing age often brings with it changes in lifestyle and health that call for some adjustments in diet. Guidelines for daily intakes of nutrients—called recommended dietary allowances (RDAs) in the United States, Recommended Nutrient Intakes (RNIs) in Canada—are broadly based. Although they do take into account the needs of men and women at different stages of life, researchers acknowledge that more studies are needed on the nutritional requirements of older adults. The body's needs may not change substantially over time, but the abilities to digest food and absorb certain nutrients diminish in older people and can cause some deficiencies.

AN ADEQUATE FLUID INTAKE

Water, which is vital for life, makes up about 60 percent of an adult body's weight. Every function, from the regulation of body temperature to digestion and elimination of waste products, requires water. Without it waste accumulates in the bloodstream and blood volume diminishes, restricting the access of oxygen and nutrients to cells. The body burns less fat and carries out almost all its functions less efficiently. Older people are more at risk for dehydration, so paying attention to fluid intake is particularly important as you age. You should drink some fluid every two to three hours, even if you don't feel thirsty. If you are concerned

THE RISK OF DEHYDRATION

Dehydration is a health concern for everyone, but the elderly are particularly at risk because they are more prone to and less able to cope with fluid deficiencies. There are many reasons for this, some of which are given below.

▶ *Sensitivity to thirst decreases, and your body may not alert you quickly enough to prevent dehydration.*

▶ *The thirst mechanism becomes less accurate as the kidneys do not reabsorb as much water before it is lost in urine.*

▶ *More fluid is lost through the skin as the skin becomes thinner with increased age.*

▶ *Elderly people may not be able to take in as much fluid from foods as they need.*

▶ *Decreased mobility or fear of incontinence may deter people from drinking as often as they would like to.*

AVOIDING THE RISK
This illustration suggests ways in which you can obtain an adequate amount of fluid throughout each day. You should try to have some liquid every two to three hours.

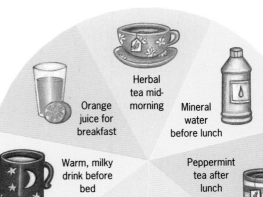

Orange juice for breakfast

Herbal tea mid-morning

Mineral water before lunch

Peppermint tea after lunch

Watery soup or broth late afternoon

Glass of fruit juice after dinner

Warm, milky drink before bed

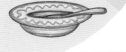

about needing to urinate during the night, have your last drink at least two hours before bedtime. Your fluid intake can include water, fruit juice, broth, herbal tea, and milk. Do not count alcohol, coffee, or regular tea as part of this intake because these are diuretics and will cause you to lose more fluid in urine. Remember too that all food contains some water; most vegetables and fruits have the highest proportion.

On the other hand, if you drink too much fluid, you may risk overhydration. The kidneys of older people do not filter as quickly as those of younger ones, which can lead to a delay in water excretion and a potentially harmful buildup of urine in the body.

AGE AND ENERGY REQUIREMENTS
It is important that your diet supply you with adequate energy—measured in calories. The body creates the energy it needs by converting the carbohydrates, protein, and fats in food to glucose, which is used as fuel.

Your metabolism—the rate at which you use energy—has started to slow down by the time you reach 40 and continues to decrease as you get older. For each decade after the age of 40, your energy requirements may decline by as much as 5 percent. This is not an inevitable consequence of aging, however, because moderate regular exercise can boost your metabolic rate by about 8 percent. If you eat more than you can burn off, you will gain weight. If this happens, it is important to scale down your calorie intake or, better still, increase your physical activity, which will help your body burn up calories, will boost your metabolic rate, and will also strengthen your bones and provide other benefits.

The nutrients required by older people are not substantially different from those needed by younger persons, but it is more important for older people to have a proper balance because their bodies are less forgiving of an unhealthy diet. Reducing your intake of such "empty calorie" foods as cookies and doughnuts, which have little nutritional value, while making sure that you have a good intake of nutrient-dense foods will help you enjoy better health.

CARBOHYDRATES
The main role of carbohydrates is to provide energy. Carbohydrates also regulate the metabolism of other nutrients,

such as protein. Regardless of age, nutritional experts suggest that you have at least six daily servings of starchy carbohydrate foods, such as bread, rice, and pasta. A serving is approximately equal to one slice of bread or 100 g (3½ ounces) of pasta.

Fiber is an important component of the diet. Soluble fiber, found in fruit, legumes, and oat bran, can help to lower high blood cholesterol, while insoluble fiber, found in whole-grain bread and brown rice, increases stool bulk and helps to prevent constipation by maintaining a healthy digestive system. From the midforties onward, a good intake of fiber—about 35 g daily—becomes especially important to prevent common complaints such as constipation.

PROTEINS
Proteins are needed by the body for maintenance and repair of the muscles, blood, organs, skin, hair, and nails. Protein is also essential for the formation of hormones and

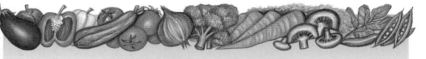

VEGETABLE LASAGNA
This recipe is an excellent source of complex carbohydrates, vitamins A and C, and calcium.

1 tbsp olive oil
1 small onion, finely chopped
175 g/6 oz mushrooms, sliced
1 red bell pepper, seeded and sliced
1 medium zucchini, sliced
225 g/8 oz can chopped tomatoes
1 tbsp chopped fresh basil
salt and freshly ground black pepper
25 g/2 tbsp butter or margarine
25 g/3 tbsp all-purpose flour
300 ml/1¼ cups low-fat (1%) milk
55 g/2 oz Cheddar cheese, grated
4 sheets precooked lasagna

■ Preheat the oven to 180°C/350°F. In a medium-size skillet, heat the olive oil over medium-high heat. Add the onions and sauté for 5 minutes or until soft. Add the mushrooms, bell pepper, and zucchini and cook, stirring, for 5 minutes.
■ Stir in the tomatoes and basil and simmer for 10 to 15 minutes. Season to taste with the salt and pepper.
■ In a small saucepan, melt the butter. Stir in the flour and cook, stirring, for 2 minutes. Slowly add the milk, stirring continuously, and bring to a boil. Cook, stirring, until thickened. Stir in the cheese.
■ Grease a 1-liter/1-quart ovenproof dish. Spoon in half the vegetable mixture and cover with 2 lasagna sheets. Spoon on half the cheese sauce. Repeat with another layer of everything. Bake for 30 minutes or until lightly browned. *Serves 2.*

YOU ARE WHAT YOU EAT

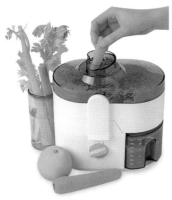

SUPER JUICER
Investing in a juicer will enable you to make fresh, healthy drinks at home and easily increase your consumption of raw fruits and vegetables.

enzymes and the efficient functioning of the immune system. In general, healthy adults should have an average daily intake of 0.8 g of protein for each kilogram (2.2 pounds) of body weight. For example, if you weigh 57 kg (125 pounds), multiply 0.8 by 57. The result is 45.6—the amount of protein you need each day. This amount can be provided by a 150 g (5½ ounce) serving of lean roast chicken; a 170 g (6 ounce) serving of poached cod fillets; or a combination of 225 g (1¼ cups) of cooked dried beans, 195 g (1 cup) of cooked brown rice, and 225 g (8 ounces) of tofu. Because all plant foods contain some protein and dairy products are rich sources, it is fairly easy to obtain sufficient protein in a varied diet.

FATS

A certain level of fat in the diet is vital for good health—for instance, to enable the absorption of the fat-soluble vitamins, A, D, E, and K, to store hormones and to provide insulation and protection for the body's inner organs. Of particular importance are the essential fatty acids (EFAs), linoleic and linolenic acid, which cannot be made by the body and must be provided by the diet.

Nuts, seeds, and polunsaturated oils, such as corn and safflower, are good sources of the essential fatty acids; so are the fats found in oily fish, like mackerel, trout, and tuna. These are beneficial in reducing the risk of heart attack, stroke, and possibly cancer. A high fat intake, however, has been linked to cardiovascular problems and the development of certain cancers; the risk of these disorders also increases with age. Therefore, your diet should consist of no more than 30 percent fat, with saturated fat limited to 10 percent. Some experts recommend even less than these amounts.

Saturated fats, found in meat, whole-milk dairy products, and coconut and palm kernel oil, contribute to high cholesterol levels. Trans-fats do the same. A by-product of the homogenization process (which makes oils solid at room temperature), trans-fats are found in many processed foods and some margarines. On the other hand, the monounsaturated fat found in olive and canola oil and the omega-3 fat in oily fish may actually help lower cholesterol levels.

VITAMINS AND MINERALS

Vitamins and minerals are essential for the efficient functioning of the body, and deficiency symptoms can develop quickly if the diet is not providing them in sufficient quantities. Vitamins A, C, and E, as well as selenium, are antioxidants, which means they help counteract the damaging effects of free radicals formed as a by-product of metabolism and are considered to have effective disease and age-fighting properties (see page 86). As people grow older, they are more prone to vitamin and mineral deficiencies because of less efficient digestion and absorption, as well as inadequate food intake (see pages 60–61).

Vitamins

Vitamin A is essential for growth, cell development, good vision, and a healthy immune system; it is also an antioxidant. Beta carotene, the plant form of vitamin A, is found in all orange, yellow, and dark green vegetables and fruits, like acorn squash, carrots, spinach, peppers, mangoes, and melon; retinol, the animal form, is found in liver, kidneys, cold-water fish, and egg yolks.

Vitamin C is thought to improve resistance to infections and reduce the damaging effects of stress. It is also required to make the protein collagen, which ensures the health of bones, teeth, and skin. In addition, vitamin C helps produce

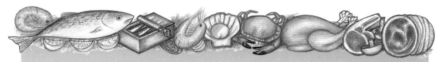

BAKED POTATO WITH TUNA AND COLESLAW

Fish is an excellent source of polyunsaturated fats. This recipe is also high in fiber and vitamins.

2 large baking potatoes
55 g/2 oz tuna in water, drained and mixed with 55 g/2 oz reduced-fat cream cheese

For the coleslaw:
115 g/4 oz green cabbage, shredded
1 medium carrot, grated
½ eating apple, cored and chopped
½ small onion, finely chopped
25 g/1 oz raisins
2 tbsp plain low-fat yogurt

■ Preheat the oven to 200°C/400°F.
■ Bake the potatoes for about

1 hour or until they feel tender when gently squeezed or poked with a fork.
■ Mix coleslaw ingredients together.
■ Cut a large cross in each potato and squeeze to enlarge the cut. Fill with the tuna mixture and serve with the coleslaw. *Serves 2.*

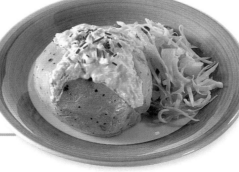

neurotransmitters, messenger chemicals that enable the body to function properly; noradrenaline, which regulates the flow of blood; and serotonin, which helps to promote sleep. Citrus fruit and fruit juices, tomatoes, kiwi fruit, strawberries, green and red peppers, and potatoes are all good sources of vitamin C. It is not stored by the body, which is why it is important to eat vitamin-C-rich fruits and vegetables every day.

Another antioxidant, vitamin E, plays a role in the health of the nervous system and in maintaining muscles and red blood cells. It is found in vegetable oils, nuts, seeds, avocados, and wheat germ.

Vitamin D, essential for healthy teeth and bones, is abundant in oily fish, egg yolks, and fortified dairy products. It can also be made by the body when the skin is exposed to sunlight; many people obtain their vitamin D in this way. The body's synthesis of vitamin D declines as we grow older, which can decrease absorption of calcium and increase the risk of osteoporosis (see page 62). It is therefore essential to obtain an adequate intake of vitamin D every day.

Vitamin K promotes normal blood clotting and is abundant in cabbage, broccoli, and other crucifers, spinach and other leafy greens, and green tea. Vitamin K is also made by bacteria in the gastrointestinal tract. If you suffer from a blood-clotting disorder, such as thrombosis, beware of eating too many foods that are rich in vitamin K. The vitamin's clotting action will reduce the effects of anticoagulant drugs.

The B vitamins—thiamine (vitamin B_1), riboflavin (B_2), niacin (B_3), pantothenic acid (B_5), pyridoxine (B_6), cobalamin (B_{12}), biotin, and folic acid (folate) are involved in releasing energy from food and making it available to the body. All are essential for adequate digestion and absorption and play a vital role in the healthy functioning of the brain, the nervous and muscular systems, and the immune system. Good sources of most of these vitamins are fortified breakfast cereals, red meat, organ meats, eggs, nuts, and legumes. Folic acid and vitamin B_{12}

DIET AND LACTOSE INTOLERANCE

Many people over 40 develop lactose intolerance—an inability to digest milk because of a deficiency of the enzyme lactase, which breaks down lactose, or milk sugar. The condition can cause discomfort, such as cramps and diarrhea. Yogurt and many cheeses cause a reaction less often in milk-sensitive individuals because the structure of lactose is changed during their production. If you cannot tolerate any milk products, other foods that are fair sources of calcium include tofu, green leafy vegetables, sesame seeds, and calcium-fortified products. The recipe below is rich in calcium and low in lactose.

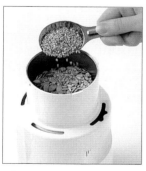

1 Grind 1 tablespoon each of sesame, pumpkin, and sunflower seeds in an electric coffee grinder.

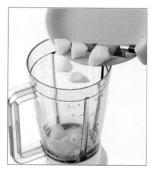

2 Blend together 4 teaspoons of the ground seeds, half a chopped mango, and 250 ml (1 cup) orange juice.

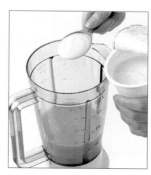

3 Add 2 tablespoons plain low-fat yogurt and blend again until a smooth liquid is produced.

4 Pour the ground seed mixture into a glass and serve. You can store the remainder in an airtight container and use it as you need it. The recipe makes about 300 ml (1¼ cups).

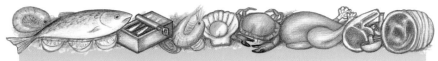

LANCASHIRE HOT POT

This recipe is rich in iron and protein and fulfills many of the necessary requirements for a healthy daily diet.

1 tbsp sunflower or canola oil
450 g/1 lb lamb stew meat, trimmed
250 g/9 oz carrots, sliced
1 large onion, chopped
pinch of sugar
salt and black pepper
1 bay leaf
1 tbsp fresh rosemary or 1 tsp dried
few sprigs parsley
25 g/1 oz pearl barley
500 g/1 lb 2 oz potatoes, thinly sliced
300 to 450 ml/1¼ to 2 cups beef or
vegetable stock or water
chopped parsley for garnish

■ Preheat the oven to 160°C/325°F.
■ In a 1-liter (1-quart) flameproof casserole, heat the oil over high heat. Add the lamb in batches and brown for about 5 minutes. Remove from the casserole and set aside.
■ Add the carrots and onion to the casserole and sauté for 5 minutes. Remove and set aside.
■ Layer the lamb and vegetables in the casserole, sprinkling with the sugar and salt and pepper to taste. Add the herbs and barley. Top with a neat layer of potatoes.
■ Add enough stock or water to come up to the potato layer. Cover and bake for 2 hours or until the meat and vegetables are tender.
■ Remove the lid, increase the oven temperature to 220°C/425°F, and bake for 20 minutes to brown the top. Garnish with the parsley. *Serves 2.*

FISH FEAST
The long life expectancy of the Japanese may be due in part to their diet, which is rich in seafood, a good source of copper, chromium, and iodine. These minerals help regulate levels of certain hormones in the body.

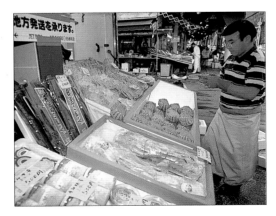

are also important to the division and growth of cells; the formation of red blood cells; and the making of DNA (a blueprint of each cell), RNA (a substance in every cell that allows it to grow and develop properly), and myelin (the sheath that surrounds nerve fibers). Folic acid and vitamin B_{12} also play important roles in the formation of proteins in the body that allow other vitamins to be absorbed. Vitamin B_{12} is found exclusively in foods of animal origin. Folic acid is abundant in many vegetables, especially the crucifers, and also in liver, legumes, avocados, yeast, and fortified cereals.

Minerals

Three minerals—sodium, potassium, and chloride—are referred to as the electrolytes; they help maintain the fluid balance in the body. Table salt is the main source of sodium and chloride in the diet. Foods rich in potassium include whole grains, bananas, citrus fruits, dried fruits, avocados, legumes, and many vegetables,

Calcium, magnesium, and phosphorus are essential for healthy bones and teeth. An adequate intake can be vital in the prevention of osteoporosis (see pages 62–63). Calcium and magnesium also assist in nerve transmission and muscle contraction. Milk products are the best sources of calcium; sardines with bones, dark leafy greens, tofu, and sesame seeds contain useful amounts too. Good sources of magnesium include leafy greens, avocados, legumes, and whole-grain cereals. Phosphorus is found in meat, egg yolks, legumes, and dairy products.

Microminerals, which include iron, copper, zinc, chromium, iodine, and selenium, are crucial to a number of body functions but are required in smaller amounts. Iron is an essential part of hemoglobin (the oxygen-carrying component in blood) and copper, which promotes iron absorption, is a component of several enzymes. Lean meat, liver, seafood, and legumes are good sources of these minerals. Older people often lack sufficient iron because they absorb it poorly. This may be due to insufficient secretion of gastric acid; heavy use of antacids, which reduce iron absorption; or bleeding caused by such medications as aspirin.

Zinc is essential for a strong immune system and wound healing; it is present in seafood, red meat, and liver. Chromium, found in whole grains, brewer's yeast, and cheese, is important for metabolizing glucose. Good sources of iodine, needed to make hormones secreted by the thyroid gland, are seafood, plant foods grown in iodine-rich soil, and iodized salt. Selenium, an important antioxidant, is found in seafood, liver, poultry, whole grains, and onions.

ANTIAGING NUTRIENTS

A healthy, well-balanced diet can do much to slow the aging process, but there are several nutrients that offer special benefits in the fight against the diseases of old age.

Many nutrients not only nourish and repair the body's systems but also help combat the processes of aging—by reducing blood cholesterol levels, for instance, strengthening the immune system, or improving metabolism or circulation.

Perhaps the most important of the antiaging nutrients are the antioxidants We know they have a beneficial effect on health, and research continues to provide more evidence of their ability to help fight disease.

ANTIOXIDANTS
As cells use oxygen to release energy from digested food, unstable molecules called free radicals are often created as a byproduct. Excessive bombardment by these molecules damages cellular DNA and other genetic material over time and may speed up aging. Antioxidants, which are believed to bind themselves to free radicals before they can cause damage, are vital to good health (see page 86 for more information).

Phytochemicals
In addition to the known antioxidants, dozens of other plant compounds, called phytochemicals, are believed to have protectice effects, and these are being studied. Two of them, genistein and indoles, are found in cruciferous vegetables, such as brussels sprouts, cabbage, and broccoli. Genistein inhibits tumor growth and indoles inhibit estrogen production, which stimulates some cancers. Isoflavones, contained in legumes, and lignans, found in flaxseeds and walnuts, also inhibit the uptake of estrogen.

Other phytochemicals include the sulfur compounds present in onions, garlic, chives, and leeks; coumaric acid and related compounds present in tomatoes, green peppers,

and carrots; lycopene in tomatoes, pink grapefruit, and watermelon; and lutein in spinach. All of these may help protect the body because of their antioxidant action or because they inhibit the formation of potentially carcinogenic substances.

THE SUPPLEMENT DEBATE
There is an ongoing debate about the value of taking nutritional supplements. While there is some evidence that getting more than the recommended amounts of particular nutrients may protect against certain degenerative diseases, it is not considered conclusive. In general, doctors warn against

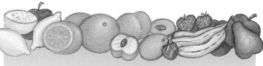

FRUIT FOOL

Peaches and apricots are both rich in beta carotene and are modest sources of vitamin C.

225 g/8 oz peaches or apricots, peeled, pitted, and sliced, or 225 g/8 oz canned fruit, drained
230 g/8 oz plain low-fat or nonfat yogurt
mint sprigs for decoration

- Reserve 4 slices of fruit for decoration and puree the rest.
- Mix the pureed fruit with the yogurt and divide the mixture between two dishes.
- Chill for 1 hour. Decorate and serve.
Serves 2.

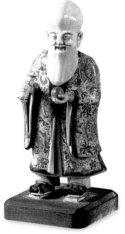

THE GOD OF LONGEVITY
In ancient Chinese mythology the peach symbolized immortality, or eternal life. Shou Lao, the god of longevity, was often depicted holding peaches. Modern research has shown that peaches have high levels of the antioxidant beta carotene.

ANTIOXIDANTS AND OTHER DISEASE FIGHTERS

Antioxidants—substances in plants that protect them against disease—may also help ward off many degenerative illnesses in humans. They include beta carotene (the precursor of vitamin A), vitamins C and E, the mineral selenium, and numerous phyto (plant) chemicals, such as bioflavonoids. Zinc also helps fight disease in its role of supporting the immune system and the action of the antioxidants. Two kinds of fat— omega-3 and monounsaturated—are important in combating heart disease and stroke because they help keep blood pressure and cholesterol at healthy levels. Omega-3 also aids in preventing blood clots.

BETA CAROTENE

Beta carotene is the plant form of the antioxidant vitamin A, which is needed for normal vision, cell division, and growth, and for healthy skin, bones, teeth, and mucous membranes. It is found in brightly colored fruits and vegetables, like sweet peppers, mangoes, carrots, and pumpkins, and also in dark green vegetables like spinach and broccoli.

VITAMIN C

Citrus fruits, kiwi fruit, tomatoes, and peppers are some of the best sources of the antioxidant vitamin C, which may protect against skin cancer. Besides its role in scavenging free radicals, vitamin C strengthens blood vessel walls; helps control cholesterol and prevent atherosclerosis; and promotes the absorption of iron.

MONOUNSATURATED FAT

The monounsaturated fat in avocados, olive oil, and canola oil can reduce the risk of heart disease and stroke by lowering LDL ("bad") cholesterol and raising HDL (("good") cholesterol. It also helps people with diabetes control their level of triglycerides.

OMEGA-3 FATTY ACIDS

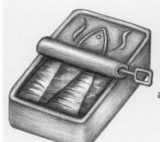

Omega-3 fatty acids, abundant in oily fish, shellfish, and flaxseeds, reduce blood pressure and cholesterol and helps prevent blood clotting, thus protecting against heart disease and stroke.

VITAMIN E

The antioxidant vitamin E prevents the harmful oxidization of fats in cell membranes. Studies have shown that it can protect the lungs against pollution and help slow the progression of Alzheimer's disease in carefully controlled doses. It is found in such plant foods as nuts, seeds, leafy greens, and vegetable oils.

ZINC

Zinc helps form the enzyme *superoxide dismutase, which* prevents cell damage. It also supports the immune system, is involved in enzyme metabolism, and is essential for growth. Important sources are nuts, shellfish, liver, and seeds.

BIOFLAVONOIDS

Bioflavonoids, which help inhibit the formation of cancer-promoting hormones, are abundant in most fresh fruits and vegetables, especially in the skins. They are also found in tea and wine. Bioflavonoids comprise just one group of the numerous plant substances known as phytochemicals, which may aid in protecting humans agains cancer and other diseases.

SELENIUM

The antioxidant mineral selenium is essential for the manufacture of the enzyme *glutathione peroxidase*, which has a significant role in neutralizing free radicals in the body. It works in tandem with vitamin E. Good sources are brazil nuts, meat, seafood, whole grains, eggs, and legumes.

taking high-dose antioxidant supplements. Some nutrients that normally act as antioxidants may actually increase oxidation. For example, high doses of vitamin C become pro-oxidant when taken by someone who has large iron reserves, and high doses of vitamin E can interfere with blood clotting, which could lead to a bleeding emergency.

It is not advisable to embark on any program of supplementation without advice from a doctor, dietitian, or nutritionist. Quantities above the recommended daily allowance, or intake, can be toxic (see box, below). It is better to obtain these nutrients through a healthy diet that includes at least five daily servings of fruits and vegetables. Also, the antioxidants are believed to work in conjunction with each other and possibly with other plant chemicals. They may not even be beneficial when taken individually.

OTHER ANTIAGING AGENTS

Ginkgo biloba has been used for thousands of years as an antiaging and digestive tonic. Ginkgo improves the blood circulation, allowing increased amounts of essential nutrients and oxygen to flow into the brain, heart, and other vital organs. Ginkgo also contains antioxidants that help protect the body from attack by free radicals. It is thought that ginkgo has an effect on the brain's chemistry, releasing more of the

A NEW LEASE ON LIFE

For over a decade Oprah Winfrey struggled to control her weight, her fluctuating size being chronicled on her TV show. When she apparently succeeded in breaking the cycle of weight gain and loss by combining a sustainable change to her eating habits with an exercise regimen, Oprah became a great example of someone who has broken the unhealthy eating patterns of a lifetime to enjoy better health.

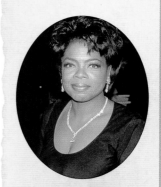

OPRAH WINFREY
Once a yo-yo dieter, Oprah has admirably fought the battle with unhealthy eating habits.

chemical serotonin, a natural painkiller that produces a feeling of well-being. However, because ginkgo acts as an anticoagulant, it should not be taken by anyone who is already taking anticlotting medication for hypertension or heart disease.

Throughout history garlic has been recognized as an important healing herb. In London in 1665 it was used in attempts to ward off the plague. In 1918 it was found to help control tuberculosis. Today herbalists and medical professionals alike recognize its health-giving and antiaging properties.

When crushed, garlic releases an enzyme called allicin, a sulfur compound that breaks down quickly in the body. This is one component responsible for the herb's antibacterial effects, making it generally useful in fighting infections. Garlic has also been shown to lower blood cholesterol and blood clotting, so it can be helpful in preventing blocked or clogged arteries. It even appears to reduce blood pressure, thus reducing the risk of strokes.

TOO MUCH OF A GOOD THING

Excessive amounts of certain nutrients can have serious effects on the body. For example, too much vitamin A can cause liver problems. High intakes of vitamin B₆ (more than 250 mg a day) can cause nerve damage, leading to loss of sensation in the hands and feet. Too much vitamin C (above 2,000 mg a day) may result in kidney stones or diarrhea. Excess vitamin D can lead to irreversible heart and kidney damage. Too much vitamin E (above 1,000 mg per day) can cause bleeding problems. Large amounts of selenium (more than 400 mcg a day) can lead to fatigue and hair loss. High intakes of potassium can result in paralysis and heart failure. Excess zinc can cause nausea, fever, and vomiting. Too much iron can damage the heart.

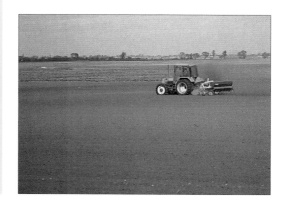

SELENIUM-RICH SOIL
The amount of selenium found in vegetables, fruits, and cereals depends on how much is present in the soil where they are grown. East Anglia is abundant in this antioxidant; interestingly, its population has the highest longevity in the United Kingdom.

DIET AND AGE-RELATED CONDITIONS

Many diseases of the past have been virtually eradicated through immunization and effective treatments. Some of the greatest threats to health in the Western world today are diet related.

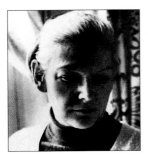

ELIZABETH DAVID
Elizabeth David introduced the Mediterranean diet to the United Kingdom, and other Western countries have discovered its virtues as well. Based largely on vegetables, fruits, fish, grains, and olive oil rather than meat, Mediterranean-style cooking has helped many people lower their risk of heart disease.

There are some health problems closely related to diet that can be effectively controlled by adjusting what you eat. In general, reducing the amount of fat in your diet, increasing your consumption of fruits and vegetables, and maintaining a stable weight suitable to your height and frame will help provide protection from many illnesses.

HIGH BLOOD PRESSURE

Blood pressure tends to rise naturally with age, but there are many other factors that can cause it to go up. All adults over age 40 should have their blood pressure checked annually—more often if high blood pressure tends to run in their family.

Because obesity increases the risk of hypertension—high blood pressure—a sensible weight reduction program can be beneficial if you are overweight. There is also good evidence that too much sodium in the diet can raise blood pressure in anyone who is sodium sensitive—perhaps as many as one in three people. Those who are susceptible should cut sodium consumption, which may reduce the need for medication. Besides not adding salt to food at the table, such people should limit their intake of

processed foods, especially bouillon cubes, instant or canned soups, chips, cheese, and smoked or cured meats.

Increasing the intake of dietary potassium, which helps balance the body's balance of fluids, can help lower blood pressure. Most plant foods contain potassium, but bananas, citrus fruits, legumes, nuts, green vegetables, avocados, tomatoes, and whole grains are particularly good sources. Some studies suggest that calcium may also help control blood pressure.

Consumption of alcohol can increase blood pressure. As few as two alcoholic drinks a day are enough to have this effect. Smoking, a sedentary lifestyle, and constant stress also contribute to hypertension.

ATHEROSCLEROSIS AND HIGH CHOLESTEROL LEVELS

Atherosclerosis—the clogging of arteries with fatty deposits—can take many decades to develop. The process occurs more rapidly, however, in smokers, the overweight, and people with high blood cholesterol levels. The hormone estrogen seems to protect women from atherosclerosis during their reproductive years because it keeps their levels of blood cholesterol low. But after menopause their risk of developing the condition equals that of men.

The most effective dietary change to prevent high cholesterol is to reduce consumption of saturated fats, which are converted to cholesterol in the body. Monounsaturated fats, such as olive and canola oil, actually decrease cholesterol levels.

Soluble fiber, found in oat and rice bran, legumes, and fruits such as apples, dried figs, and apricots, helps reduce blood cholesterol by binding to it in the small intes-

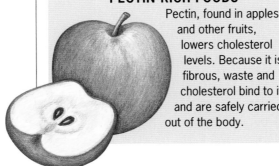

PECTIN-RICH FOODS
Pectin, found in apples and other fruits, lowers cholesterol levels. Because it is fibrous, waste and cholesterol bind to it and are safely carried out of the body.

tine and preventing its reabsorption by the body. The bound cholesterol is then excreted. A diet high in fruits and vegetables also provides plenty of antioxidants (see pages 85–86), which may offer some protection against atherosclerosis.

CANCER

Many scientists believe that at least one-third of all cancers are diet related. Certain dietary elements apparently help promote the development and spread of malignancies, while others seem to slow or block them. Fat is one of the culprits; it may increase the risk of cancers of the colon, uterus, prostate, and skin. It is advisable to limit total fat intake to less than 30 percent of total calories (some experts believe that 20 percent is even better) and keep the intake of saturated fat at 10 percent or less.

A high intake of beta carotene (the plant form of vitamin A) has been associated with lower rates of lung cancer. Vitamin C, which seems to block carcinogens in the stomach, may decrease the risk of stomach cancer. The high fiber content of fruits and vegetables is also thought to be beneficial.

More than 200 studies worldwide have found that a high consumption of fruits, vegetables, and whole grains increases resistance to several cancers, including cancer of the breast, mouth, esophagus, stomach, lung, and prostate. In addition to the antioxidants, fruits and vegetables also contain compounds called phytochemicals, which appear to decrease the risk of certain cancers by stimulating enzymes that block carcinogens from penetrating body cells.

OSTEOPOROSIS

Osteoporosis, or bone-wasting disease, is a major cause of bone fractures in the elderly (see pages 62–63). A high intake of calcium throughout adolescence and young adulthood can help prevent this disease in later life by strengthening the bones.

Some health experts advise postmenopausal women and men over 65 to have a daily calcium intake of 1,200 to 1,500 mg. Dairy products, legumes, canned fish with bones, green leafy vegetables, and tofu are all good sources of calcium. However, certain kinds of fiber, found especially in legumes, nuts, and whole grains, can decrease the amount of calcium absorbed because of the presence of

phytates (phytic acid). Oxalates in dark leafy greens, rhubarb, beets, berries, and grapes also decrease absorption of calcium. In order to absorb calcium effectively, the body also needs vitamin D (see page 83) either from sunlight or from dietary sources.

DIABETES AND HYPOGLYCEMIA

To reduce the risk of developing diabetes, you need a diet low in sugar and other refined carbohydrates and high in fiber. It is also important to maintain a weight healthy for your height and age—adult-onset diabetes is more prevalent in the obese. Diabetics are particularly prone to heart disease, so a diet low in saturated fats and high in monunsaturated fats is vital. This approach will benefit you whether you suffer from diabetes or not.

Keeping a stable blood sugar level is an important element in controlling diabetes. hypoglycemia (low blood sugar) can result when glucose levels plummet and can lead to coma or even death. Hyperglycemia, in which the glucose in the blood is too high, can also be very dangerous. Starchy foods such as bread, pasta, and rice are broken

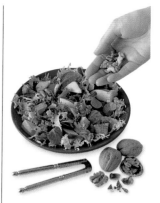

THE WONDER OF WALNUTS
A study reported in the New England Journal of Medicine *found that walnuts are an effective way of lowering blood cholesterol levels. People who ate about 25 g (1 oz) of walnuts a week had 10 percent lower cholesterol than those who did not.*

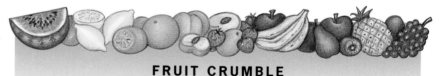

FRUIT CRUMBLE

This delicious crumble provides a healthy amount of fiber, which helps to lower high cholesterol levels.

225 g/8 oz cooking apples, peeled, cored, and chopped
225 g/8 oz plums, halved and pitted
40–55 g/3–4 tbsp granulated sugar
55 g/⅓ cup whole-wheat flour
25 g/3 tbsp all-purpose flour
55 g/4 tbsp butter
55 g/¼ cup brown sugar
25 g/1 oz oatmeal

■ Preheat the oven to 190°C/375°F
■ Arrange the fruit in a 600-ml/2-cup ovenproof dish and sprinkle the granulated sugar over it.
■ Sift the flours into a bowl, rub in the butter until the mixture resembles fine bread crumbs, and stir in the brown sugar and oatmeal.
■ Sprinkle the crumble evenly over the fruit. Bake for 20 to 30 minutes or until the fruit is soft and the topping crisp.
■ Serve with custard or plain low-fat yogurt if desired.
Serves 2.

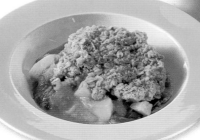

down more slowly in the gut and consequently do not cause the rapid rise in blood sugar levels that refined carbohydrates do.

The mineral chromium is important in regulating blood sugar levels and also helps regulate blood cholesterol levels. Rich sources of chromium include liver, whole-grain cereals, and cheese.

ARTHRITIS

Rheumatoid arthritis (see page 65) can affect people of all ages and is more common in women than men. Arthritis is more painful if you are overweight because the extra weight places more strain on the weight-bearing joints.

Certain types of polyunsaturated fats called omega-3 fatty acids have been shown to decrease inflammation in the joints of rheumatoid arthritis sufferers. Omega-3 fatty acids are present in oily fish, such as salmon, trout, mackerel, sardines, and herring. Including two portions of oily fish in the weekly diet may help decrease the inflammation. Fish oil supplements and evening primrose oil have a similar effect but should be used only if recommended and monitored by a doctor or dietitian.

A diet high in fruits and vegetables is also thought to benefit rheumatoid arthritis sufferers because it may prevent the bacteria in the large bowel from multiplying rapidly. Bowel bacteria are thought to cause the immune system to overreact.

Osteoarthritis develops with age when the cartilage of the joint deteriorates. Obese people are more likely to suffer from osteoarthritis because their excess weight puts undue stress on the joints. A healthy low-fat diet, combined with gentle exercise, can help prevent or relieve osteoarthritis.

MENOPAUSAL SYMPTOMS

A decrease in estrogen after menopause can increase the risk of developing osteoporosis and heart disease. Dietary measures to minimize this risk, as discussed above, are vital. A low-fat diet is particularly beneficial at this stage because many menopausal women are more susceptible to weight gain.

Phytoestrogens, which mimic the female hormone estrogen, are abundant in soy products (but not soy sauce) and have been linked to a reduced risk of coronary heart disease and certain forms of breast cancer in older women. They also reduce the severity of menopausal symptoms.

CONSTIPATION

The elderly are particularly prone to constipation, which can result from decreased muscle tone in the gastrointestinal tract and a low-fiber diet combined with a low fluid intake. Constipation is a common condition that has been linked to many diseases, including cancer of the large bowel. Insoluble fiber helps to prevent constipation by increasing stool bulk, thus promoting regular bowel movements. Eat plenty of whole-grain bread and cereals and unpeeled fruit, which are all rich in insoluble fiber. A fluid intake of at least eight glasses a day prevents dehydration and makes stools easier to expel. Regular physical activity can also stimulate bowel movements.

SIGHT PROBLEMS

The chief cause of poor vision and blindness in people over 50 is macular degeneration, which occurs when the central part of the retina deteriorates. Eating too much saturated fat is thought to make people more

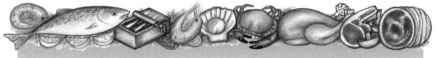

SALMON STEAK WITH PESTO SAUCE

Salmon is an excellent source of omega-3 fatty acids, helpful for combating the painful joints of arthritis.

2 tsp olive oil plus some for coating the foil
2 salmon steaks, about
   175 g/6 oz each
2 sprigs fresh dill
1/2 a lemon
salt and freshly ground black pepper
1 tbsp pesto sauce
115 g/4 oz plain low-fat yogurt

■ Preheat the oven to 180°C/350°F. Brush 2 sheets of foil with olive oil.
■ Place a salmon steak in the center of each piece of foil, lay a sprig of dill on each steak, and squeeze lemon juice over all of them. Drizzle with the 2 tsp of olive oil and season with salt and pepper to taste.
■ Wrap the foil around the salmon to form a parcel. Bake for 20 minutes.
■ Meanwhile, make the sauce. In a small saucepan over low heat, stir together the pesto sauce and yogurt until hot but not bubbling.
■ Remove the salmon from the foil and serve immediately with the sauce, new potatoes, and green beans. *Serves 2.*

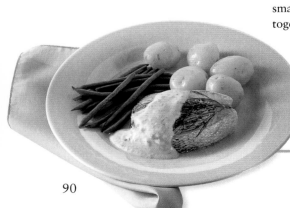

THE MENOPAUSE DIET

Hormonal changes that occur during menopause make your body less efficient at metabolizing certain vitamins and minerals. Eating foods rich in the nutrients lost may help to lessen any symptoms and prevent disease.

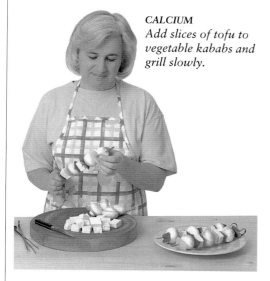

CALCIUM
Add slices of tofu to vegetable kababs and grill slowly.

If your diet contains the following foods on a regular basis, you may find menopause easier to deal with.

▶ *Milk,tofu curded with calcium salts,leafy greens, and canned sardines with bones contain calcium to lower the risk of osteoporosis.*

▶ *Whole grains, green vegetables, nuts, and seeds contain magnesium, which helps the body use calcium and vitamin D efficiently.*

▶ *Soybeans and soy products contain phytoestrogens, which can help ease many menopausal symptoms and may also protect against osteoporosis.*

▶ *Avocados, nuts, and leafy greens contain vitamin E, which may help relieve some menopausal symptoms.*

susceptible to the condition. A 10-year study of 2,000 men and women aged 45 to 84 at the University of Wisconsin Medical School found that early signs of macular degeneration were 80 percent more common in persons with a diet high in saturated fat than in those who ate little fat. This may be due to fat-clogged arteries restricting blood flow to the retina or fat in the retina blocking nutrients from cells. Cataracts, another common sight problem associated with age, are now believed to be significantly related to the intake of antioxidants. Eating plenty of foods containing vitamins A, C, and E can reduce your risk of developing them.

ALCOHOL AND YOUR HEALTH
Certain forms of alcohol, such as red wine, are known to contain substances that can benefit health. There is evidence from many clinical studies that people who drink alcohol—especially wine—in moderation enjoy some protection against coronary heart disease. Alcohol also stimulates the appetite and promotes relaxation.

Too much alcohol is harmful, however, and its effects may be even worse for older people, who have a diminished ability to process it. Alcohol widens the small blood vessels of the skin, making it become flushed.

Because it is an appetite stimulant, it may also encourage some people to eat too much, leading to obesity. Alcohol is a diuretic as well and can increase the risk of dehydration, which is already a problem for older people (see page 80). The toxic effects of prolonged heavy use of alcohol can also cause brain damage. Very heavy drinkers may suffer from alcoholic dementia. Other effects of excessive alcohol include liver damage, anemia, high blood pressure, pancreas damage, and heart muscle damage.

Medical recommendations for a safe intake of alcohol are one unit per day for women and two per day for men. One unit of alcohol is equivalent to a 175 or 200 ml (4- or 5-ounce) glass of wine, 500 ml (12 ounces) of beer, or a 30-ml (1½-ounce) measure of spirits.

EAT YOUR GREENS
It is the brightly colored carotenoids in vegetables that benefit your sight. These carotenoids are also present in leafy green vegetables like spinach but are hidden by the chlorophyll.

Preventing mascular degeneration
There is evidence that a high intake of certain vegetables significantly reduces the risk of developing one type of macular degeneration. The beneficial agents appear to be two carotenoids: lutein, and zeaxanthin, which are present in the yellow, orange, and red pigments of plant foods. Vegetables that contain these carotenoids include sweet peppers, corn, and such leafy green vegetables as spinach.

CHANGING EATING HABITS

As people advance in years, their eating habits may change for many reasons. They could be at greater risk for nutritional deficiencies as a result.

Many factors can affect diet as a person grows older. Physical changes, such as a deterioration in taste, smell, or mobility, and lifestyle changes, such as altered income, may result in poor food intake or a diet lacking in some essential nutrients. This can be a serious problem for older people; they may become more prone to illness resulting from a poor diet. Eating badly can diminish physical strength, decrease the efficiency of the immune system, and hinder the body's ability to heal itself.

THE EFFECT OF AGE ON APPETITE, TASTE, AND SMELL

A lower rate of activity and energy expenditure in older people may result in a diminished appetite. This, in turn, may lead to a reduced intake of essential nutrients, as well as excessive weight loss, which can be dangerous for the elderly. Becoming more physically active is a good appetite stimulant. Also, drinking a bitter herbal tea like gentian root can help improve appetite because it increases the flow of saliva and stomach juices.

The sense of taste can change gradually over the years (see page 72). The number of active tastebuds declines as you age, and your sense of smell may also decrease as the lining of mucous membranes in the nose becomes thinner and less sensitive. Habitual smoking can reduce the perception of specific tastes and it may also impair the ability to smell.

A decline in the sense of taste can lead to a lack of interest in food or excessive use of flavor enhancers such as sugar and salt. It's better to use more herbs and spices rather than sugar or salt; they can dramatically improve the flavor of food, and some will provide other health benefits as well (see page 93). For example, adding fresh cilantro to a stir-fry will stimulate your appetite while providing flavor. Seasonings like horseradish, which stimulate the nasal aspect of taste, are often more appreciated as people grow older.

Loss of teeth or weakening of gums (see page 149) in older people may lead to eating a smaller variety of foods, which can result in nutritional deficiencies. And an inability to chew properly or eat tough food may cause people to choose soft foods pri-

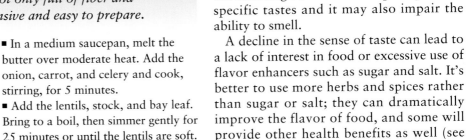

CARROT AND LENTIL SOUP

This homemade soup is not only full of fiber and nutrients but also is inexpensive and easy to prepare.

15 g/1 tsbp butter or margarine
115 g/4 oz (1 small) onion, chopped
115 g/4 oz (1 large) carrot, chopped
1 stalk celery, chopped
55 g/2 oz red lentils
600 ml/2½ cups vegetable or chicken stock, skimmed of fat
1 bay leaf
salt and freshly ground black pepper
chopped fresh parsley for garnish

■ In a medium saucepan, melt the butter over moderate heat. Add the onion, carrot, and celery and cook, stirring, for 5 minutes.
■ Add the lentils, stock, and bay leaf. Bring to a boil, then simmer gently for 25 minutes or until the lentils are soft.
■ Remove the bay leaf and puree the soup in a food processor or blender.
■ Reheat; add salt and pepper to taste.
■ Serve garnished with parsley and accompanied by whole-wheat rolls.
Serves 2.

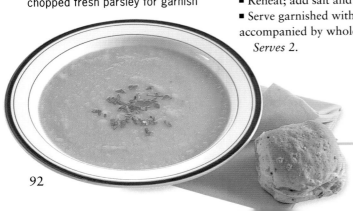

HERBS AND SPICES FOR HEALTH

If you have a diminishing sense of taste, it can help to familiarize yourself with the culinary benefits of herbs and spices. There is a wide range of aromatic herbs and spices available, and many of these will not only flavor your food but also protect your health. Below is just a small sampling.

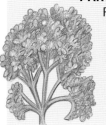

PARSLEY
Parsley provides vitamins A and C and several minerals. Use the herb with any savory dish.

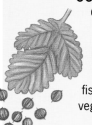

CORIANDER
Coriander cleanses and benefits the urinary tract. Add this spice to curries and to fish, chicken, and vegetable dishes.

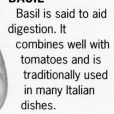

DILL
Dill can help relieve flatulence. It enhances salads and cheese and fish dishes.

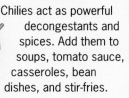

CHILIES
Chilies act as powerful decongestants and spices. Add them to soups, tomato sauce, casseroles, bean dishes, and stir-fries.

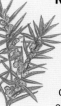

ROSEMARY
Rosemary is thought to help circulation and the digestive system. It is especially good with lamb and potato dishes.

BASIL
Basil is said to aid digestion. It combines well with tomatoes and is traditionally used in many Italian dishes.

marily, leading to insufficient fiber in the diet and to digestion and bowel problems. If you suffer from mouth and teeth problems, consider investing in a food processor or blender. With this appliance you can make easy-to-eat nutritious soups, pâtés, sauces, and nourishing drinks using fresh ingredients. However, it is also important to seek the advice of a dentist so that you can continue to eat whole foods. If food is not chewed, it is not mixed with enough saliva. This in itself can cause problems because saliva plays an important role in the digestive process. Without it, extra demands are placed on the stomach.

Medications can also affect appetite; some will depress it, while others may stimulate it and lead to overeating. Still others will affect taste. If you are taking any medication on a regular basis and think it could be adversely affecting your eating habits, ask your doctor for advice.

SOCIAL EFFECTS ON EATING HABITS
Many elderly people living alone may not have a sufficiently varied diet. This might be due to impaired mobility or simply to lack of motivation to prepare meals for one person. After all, food is not just for nutrition; it serves a social, psychological, and cultural function, and when these functions are no longer part of the picture, the desire to eat may decrease markedly. Some of the pleasure of eating comes from cooking with or for another person and then sitting down to

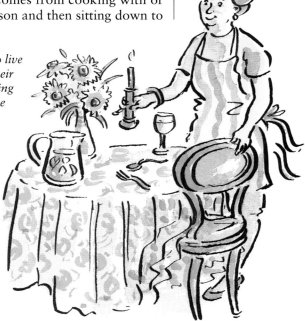

Solo eating
Some people who live alone find that their diet suffers. Making an effort to set the table attractively and cook well-balanced meals for yourself every day is a healthy habit to develop.

Kitchen Garden

Growing your own fresh garden produce is doubly rewarding. It not only enriches your diet with foods that are full of flavor and many essential nutrients needed for a healthy life but also gives you a well-earned sense of achievement.

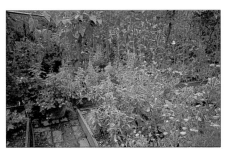

GROWING YOUR OWN
Every home used to have a kitchen garden if there was room for one. There is no better way to ensure the freshness of your food.

A vegetable plot can be an attractive and practical addition to your garden. Raised beds will maximize available growing space and are a good idea if you suffer from back problems. Compact, trailing varieties of fruits and vegetables can be trained to tumble down the sides, giving you more space for planting in the beds themselves. Tomatoes and strawberries grow particularly well this way. Compact varieties can also be grown in containers if you don't have a garden plot.

CONTAINER GARDENING

Try planting containers with "cut and come again" crops of vegetables such as mesclun mix lettuce. You will get three crops if you snip greens as soon as they are about 4 inches high. Combinations of plants in the same container can make an interesting focal point while saving space. Strawberries and spring lettuces work especially well; sweet peas and runner beans can be grown on supports in the same container.

STORING YOUR CROP

One problem with garden fruits and vegetables is that the whole crop tends to be ready at one time. The following can be frozen: asparagus, berries, broccoli, brussels sprouts, carrots, cauliflower, green beans, leeks, peas, and spinach. Vegetables must be blanched before freezing them.

STORING PRODUCE
Proper storage will ensure that you enjoy the fruits of your hard work for months to come.

MAKING YOUR OWN FERTILIZER

The better the growing conditions for vegetables, the more bountiful your crop is likely to be. The key is to water them often and provide them with plenty of fertilizer. To keep costs down, make your own fertilizer from nettles and any weeds that have not gone to seed.

1 *Press fresh nettle or weed leaves into a container. Add about 10 liters (2½ gallons) of water for every 1 kg (2.2 lb) of leaves. Stir; cover with plastic wrap.*

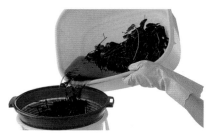

2 *Leave the mixture for about eight weeks. Strain it and dilute with 10 parts water before using. Use the remains of the leaves as compost.*

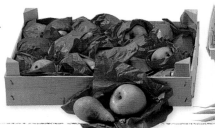

Apples and pears can be wrapped in paper and stored in a cool, well-ventilated place. Ideally, fruits should not touch each other.

Carrots, rutabagas, and turnips can be stored in boxes of cool, dry sand.

Onions should be dried and hung up in nets.

conversation and company. This may be one of the reasons that many widowed people lose the incentive to eat proper meals. Of course, bereavement, depression, and loneliness can also decrease appetite. Conversely, in times of crisis, many people turn to familiar foods for comfort because they represent warmth and security. Anxiety, boredom, and loneliness can also lead to unhealthy eating patterns.

People who do not like to eat alone should find opportunities to share meals, for both psychological and nutritional health. Some groups organize community meals for older people, but having a circle of friends with whom to share meals is also important. The meals do not have to be complicated. Just sharing a simple dish of pasta and a salad or having a regular pot-luck event to which each person brings a dish can be enjoyable and easy to prepare for.

Joining a social or sports club or association can give you an opportunity to make new friends and become involved in regular activities. You might even choose to take a cooking course in which you can gain new ideas on food preparation. You could also establish a regular time to share a meal with

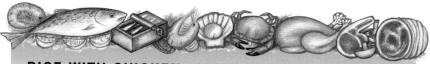

RICE WITH CHICKEN, ONIONS, AND MUSHROOMS

This dish is easy, flavorful, and economical. Add a salad and you have three of your daily vegetable servings in one meal.

1 tbsp olive oil
55 g/2 oz bacon, chopped
1 small onion, chopped
1 leek, chopped
½ red bell pepper, seeded and chopped
115 g/4 oz mushrooms, chopped
115 g/4 oz (⅔ cup) long-grain rice
175 g/6 oz cooked chicken, diced
225 g/8 oz can chopped tomatoes
200 ml/7 fl oz chicken stock
1 tbsp chopped parsley, plus extra for garnish
salt and black pepper to taste

■ In a medium saucepan, heat the oil over high heat. Add the bacon and sauté, stirring, until browned. Add the onion, leek, red pepper, and mushrooms; cook, stirring, until soft.

■ Add the rice and cook, stirring, for approximately 1 minute.
■ Stir in all the remaining ingredients. Bring to a boil, cover, and simmer for 20 minutes or until all the liquid has been absorbed.
■ Serve with a mixed salad.
Serves 2.

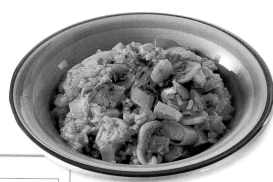

MAINTAINING HEALTHY EATING PATTERNS

Although most people understand the importance of healthy eating, it may be daunting to change long-standing poor habits. More often than not, however, a dramatic change is not necessary. It is relatively simple to include more nutritious and low-fat foods in your diet without making your mealtimes time-consuming or expensive. Try some of the suggestions given below.

▶ *Use nonfat or low-fat milk instead of regular milk.*

▶ *Buy low-fat or nonfat versions of cheese, yogurt, mayonnaise, salad dressing, and sour cream.*

▶ *Eat less red meat and more fish, white meat of poultry, and legumes.*

▶ *Switch from white to whole-grain bread; this will give you more nutrients and fiber.*

▶ *Buy fresh or frozen fruit to eat for desserts.*

▶ *Choose unsweetened juices and canned fruit preserved in juice rather than syrup.*

▶ *Use strong-tasting cheeses such as Roquefort, Stilton, Romano, and Parmesan in cooking to add flavor with less cheese.*

▶ *Look for low-salt versions of food and use more herbs and spices for flavor.*

SAVE THE BOUNTY
If you have a surfeit of apples, pears, or other fruit, cut them up and stew them in a little water. Once they have cooled, freeze them and use them later for desserts or condiments.

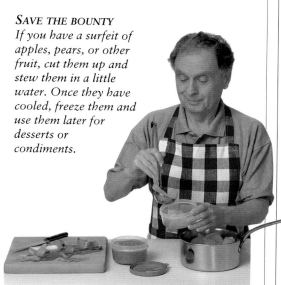

STORING AND PREPARING FOOD

Preparing and storing food properly is important both for safety and for preserving nutrients.

▶ *Use fresh fruits and vegetables as soon as possible after buying them. The longer you store them, the more nutrients they lose.*

▶ *If you do not shop often, buy frozen fruits and vegetables; they are sometimes even more nutritious than fresh products because they are picked at their peak and frozen soon afterward.*

▶ *Cook fruits and vegetables for as brief a time as possible and eat them as soon as they are ready.*

FREEZER LABELS
When you are packing food for freezing, make sure that you label and date each item. This not only is useful for identification but also lets you know when the food should be eaten.

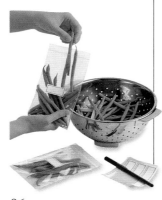

relatives—their place or yours. Let them know how much it means to you. Creating the right atmosphere for enjoying your food is an important part of ensuring that you maintain a healthy diet.

ECONOMIC FACTORS

A reduced income is often an obstacle to eating properly. Trying to make ends meet may mean that food takes a low priority, while decreased mobility may result in shopping at closer but more expensive stores rather than going to a more distant supermarket where the prices are better and the selection of food greater.

There are several ways in which you can get the best nutrition for the least amount of money. For example, most supermarkets have weekly specials. Take advantage of these buys, even if you can't use some of the products right away. You can freeze fresh foods for future use (see page 94 for fruits and vegetables that are suitable for freezing) and keep canned and packaged foods on your pantry shelf for up to a year. For convenience, slice bread and divide other foods for freezing into meal-size portions.

Buy fruits and vegetables when they are in season; they are less expensive and more nutritious. They are also less likely to have been stored for long periods and will therefore be fresher. Roadside and farmer's markets are good sources of seasonal fruits and vegetables and their prices are often less than those at a supermarket.

Take advantage of bulk buys if you can. They do require a greater outlay of cash in the short term, but they will save you money in the long run. If you cannot afford to buy in bulk for yourself or you don't have the storage space, see if you can team up with a friend or relative to share items.

To get the best buys in carbohydrates like rice, bread, and breakfast cereal, always go for whole-grain rather than refined versions. These not only provide more nutrients but also contain more of the fiber you need.

Even if you should find yourself with more disposable income in your later years, following the above advice is still sensible. With the money you save, you can enjoy more meals out and occasionally splurge on more expensive foods. It is still important to keep an eye on diet, however, because you could be eating food that is too high in fat or salt or drinking too much alcohol.

FOOD SAFETY

Foods must be stored and cooked properly so that they do not develop harmful microorganisms. Food poisoning, which may result from improper storage or cooking, can seriously debilitate older people. Make sure that your kitchen is clean and that you never keep food too long or eat food that is past its "use by" date.

Cook meat, poultry, eggs, and fish thoroughly before you eat them. All parts of the food must be heated to at least 75°C (167°F) to destroy bacteria. Elderly people should not eat meat that is rare or raw eggs, as in homemade mayonnaise.

It is better to defrost frozen poultry, fish, and meat in the refrigerator or microwave oven rather than on the countertop. The outside of the food may develop bacteria before the inside has thawed.

Bacteria need warmth, moisture, and nutrients to thrive, all of which can be amply provided by a warm kitchen. Food hygienists advise keeping cold foods cold and hot foods hot; they should not be left standing at room temperature for more than two hours. The one exception is any food that is preserved in an acid medium, such as vinegar or lemon juice.

CHECKLIST
The following tips will help you keep your food free from germs and harmful bacteria:

✔ *Wash hands thoroughly before and after food preparation.*

✔ *Prepare food as close to the time of eating as possible.*

✔ *Store leftovers promptly and use them within two days. Reheat food, especially meat, only once.*

✔ *Store different foods separately to avoid cross contamination.*

✔ *Wash all implements and dishes in the hottest water possible soon after they are used.*

✔ *Never use foods past their "use by" date or any that look or smell spoiled.*

✔ *After using a cutting board for meat, fish, or poultry, scrub the board and knives thoroughly.*

CHAPTER 5

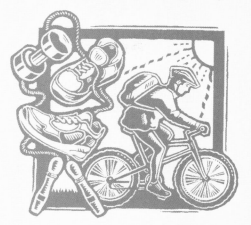

STAYING PHYSICALLY ACTIVE

As you grow older, the need to keep active becomes increasingly important. Exercise will help prevent some of the effects of aging not only on your body but on your mind as well, enabling you to maintain an independent and enjoyable lifestyle and slowing down the aging process.

THE IMPORTANCE OF EXERCISE

It is never too late to start an exercise program. A combination of aerobic, strength, and stretching exercises can be beneficial to your quality of life, as well as your fitness.

A sedentary lifestyle increases the risk of developing orthopedic problems, heart disease, and even some cancers. By exercising regularly, even if you start late in life, you can maintain a strong, supple body while protecting yourself from a range of disorders. Most experts agree that doing vigorous exercise regularly is one of the most important ways in which you can hold back the clock.

IT'S NEVER TOO LATE

If you have been inactive and remain so in later life, you could be putting yourself in danger of spending the last few years of your life diseased and virtually immobilized. A nine-year study at the Cooper Clinic in Dallas, Texas, showed that people who exercise regularly not only live longer than those who are sedentary but also spend less money on doctor visits and hospital stays.

Exercise is beneficial at any age, regardless of how sedentary you have previously been, even if 10 or more years have passed since you exercised regularly. Studies have shown that people in their eighties and nineties with mobility problems can quickly build muscle strength and size with weight training. In 1988 at Tufts University in Massachusetts, Dr. William Evans found that men between 60 and 72 years of age increased their muscle mass by an average of 15 percent and their muscle strength by 200 percent with regular exercise and weight training.

This optimistic evidence is supported by a National Fitness Survey in the United Kingdom published in 1990, which found that elderly people could be as fit as or fitter than some adults 10 or more years younger. In fact, many changes in mobility attributed to aging are caused by lack of activity and therefore can be corrected by activity.

Experts have concluded that regular exercise not only prolongs life but also delays disability. Studies have established that inactive individuals over the age of 55 fall or injure themselves more often than those who are active, and individuals who have maintained both muscle tone and mobility will stumble rather than fall.

A 1997 survey revealed that 63 percent of Canadians are not active enough to sustain good health. To deal with the problem Health Canada and other health and fitness organizations produced the Physical Activity Guide to Healthy Active Living. It recommends 30 to 60 minutes of daily activity— for example, taking the stairs instead of an elevator or walking at least part of the distance to work or an appointment—that can be added up in periods of 10 minutes each.

continued on page 102

A NEW LEASE ON LIFE

On his 95th birthday (he was born in 1902) Everitt Hosack broke a world long-jump record in the 75- to 100-year-old category and won five gold medals at the European Indoor Veterans Athletics championships. Although American, Everitt was allowed to compete in the European games because he was the only athlete in the 90- to 100-year-old group. Everitt gave up sports for over 50 years before returning to excel in the long jump, high jump, 60-meter, 400-meter, and shot-put events.

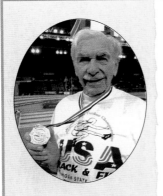

EVERGREEN CHAMPION
Even at the age of 95, Everitt Hosack begins every day with a jog to keep himself fit.

THE HEALTH BENEFITS OF EXERCISE

Although some decline will take place, your body is not a machine that will inevitably wear out because it has the capability to repair and renew itself. And if taken care of properly, it even has the capacity to become stronger and fitter. With improper care the inevitable changes that occur may threaten your independence and mobility. However, regular exercise will provide you with manifold benefits, not just for your body but for your emotional well-being as well. In some respects exercise can reverse the effects of a poor and sedentary lifestyle. A few of the health benefits of getting moving are listed below.

MIND POWER
Exercise improves your blood flow, allowing you to concentrate better and enhancing your memory and mental alertness. You will also sleep more soundly. A 12-year study of 6,500 elderly people, conducted by Professor P. Rabbit at Manchester University, England, and published in 1995, showed that very fit 70-year-olds have the mental abilities of people 20 years younger.

SKIN
Exercise increases blood flow to the skin, permitting adequate amounts of nutrients and oxygen to reach it and keep it healthy. Toxins in the blood are also flushed out when you sweat during exercise. And the increased blood flow to the dermis (see page 141) allows your skin to repair itself more efficiently if it is injured.

DIGESTION
Exercise increases blood flow to the digestive system, which makes the absorption of nutrients into the blood more efficient. The muscles of the digestive system also benefit from exercise, which in turn can help to prevent or relieve constipation and diverticulosis and also reduce the likelihood of hiatal hernia, which is a potential problem for older people.

SEX LIFE
Exercise makes you feel more refreshed and confident about your body and can also improve your sex drive, flexibility, and stamina. Men who exercise regularly find it easier to achieve and maintain erections, and healthy women find it easier to reach arousal and orgasm.

BALANCE
The strengthening of muscles and bones as you exercise will benefit your balance and coordination. This in turn will allow you to remain mobile and independent as you grow older. Good balance means that the likelihood of falls and injuries is dramatically reduced. Balance also allows you to do more exercise, so that the benefits you gain are constantly increasing.

STAMINA
Regular aerobic activity will help to maintain the elasticity of your lungs, enabling them to take in more oxygen and exchange oxygen and carbon dioxide more efficiently. This ensures that an adequate amount of oxygen reaches your blood and thus increases your stamina, so that you get more out of your daily life without being dogged by tiredness.

BONES AND JOINTS
Because your bones are strengthened and become denser as you exercise, they are less likely to become brittle or ache as you age, and you are less likely to succumb to osteoporosis (see page 62). Exercise also keeps your joints mobile. For optimum benefit you should put each joint ithrough its full range of movement regularly.

CARDIOVASCULAR HEALTH
Regular aerobic exercise improves the health of your heart and circulation and effectively lowers your blood pressure and cholesterol levels. A one-year study of previously sedentary men showed that running 12 to 16 km (8 to 10 miles) a week significantly increased the levels of high-density lipoproteins, or "good'" cholesterol, in their blood.

STRESS
Exercise is an effective way to relieve the physical, hormonal, and emotional effects of stress, thus reducing the likelihood of developing a stress-related illness. Exercise also acts as an anti-depressant because it stimulates the release of endorphins, natural painkillers, in the brain. Studies have shown that those who lead sedentary lives report more anxiety.

MUSCLES
Exercising your muscles improves your strength and flexibility. More muscle bulk in proportion to fat also increases your metabolic rate (see page 102) and insulin sensitivity (see page 103) and helps control weight. The stronger your muscles, the more likely it is that you will be able to remain independent into old age.

Gardening

Getting Fit with

You don't necessarily have to take up a sport to become fit. A physical hobby like gardening can provide the same benefits to your health. You are also more likely to exercise regularly if you are involved in an activity that you enjoy.

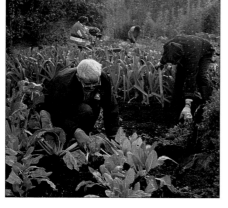

GARDENING FOR ALL
If you don't have a garden but enjoy working with plants, there are plenty of opportunities to do so. Historic homes often need volunteers to help take care of their grounds. You could also apply for a plot in a community garden.

Gardening is a popular pastime among people of all ages and is an excellent way to increase activity levels. The fresh air will improve your respiratory health, and exposure to natural light will increase levels of vitamin D, which many older people lack. Gardening is also good exercise, burning up a surprising number of calories. The process of growing and nurturing plants is good for your emotional health too and provides a purpose throughout the year. But it is important to protect yourself from the elements when in the garden by wearing a sunscreen in the summer and wrapping up well on cold days.

GOOD LIFTING TECHNIQUE

Your back is a vitally important structure. Look after it by lifting things properly: keep your back straight, bend your knees, and let your legs do the work. Use this method when you are bending to lift anything, even your gardening gloves or a few cut flowers. If you are stiff, use a tool—such as a fork plunged in the ground—to help you move.

WARMING UP AND COOLING DOWN

Gardening can be strenuous, and you may feel very stiff or even injure yourself if you do not warm up first and cool down afterward. Before you start, stretch your arms and back by reaching up as high as you can and then swing your arms around. Sit on a chair and stretch your legs out in front of you; hold the pose for a count of eight. Walk around the garden a few times before beginning work. Repeat these exercises after you have finished a gardening session, to wind down, and then treat yourself to a soothing bath.

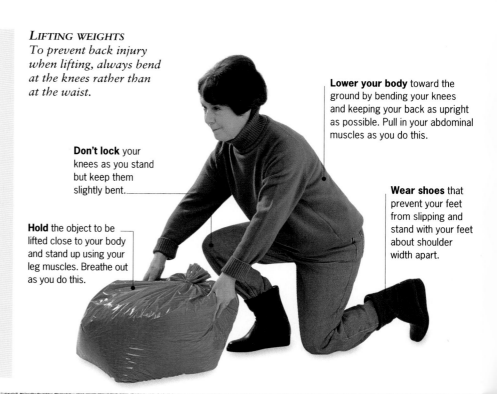

LIFTING WEIGHTS
To prevent back injury when lifting, always bend at the knees rather than at the waist.

Don't lock your knees as you stand but keep them slightly bent.

Hold the object to be lifted close to your body and stand up using your leg muscles. Breathe out as you do this.

Lower your body toward the ground by bending your knees and keeping your back as upright as possible. Pull in your abdominal muscles as you do this.

Wear shoes that prevent your feet from slipping and stand with your feet about shoulder width apart.

COMMON GARDEN JOBS

Gardening is an all-round fitness activity. The bending and stretching involved improve flexibility, and digging, carrying watering cans, and turning compost help increase

strength. Your stamina will also benefit, provided you work steadily for at least half an hour. Examples of gardening activities that make effective exercises are shown here.

RAKING LEAVES
Raking is an excellent stretching exercise if you make an effort to reach forward while you are working. Vigorous raking will burn up about 120 calories in 40 to 45 minutes.

Trim your waist by gently twisting your body.

Remember to keep your back straight.

TRIMMING A HEDGE
Reaching up to trim a hedge will improve the strength of your arms and upper body and also increase your flexibility and stamina. On average, hedge clipping will use up about 120 calories in 40 minutes.

PUSHING A WHEELBARROW
Wheeling items around your garden will provide you with upper body exercise, as well as improve your stamina. If you use the wheelbarrow regularly, you will burn extra calories. Keep your body straight.

Posture should be upright; use your legs, buttocks, and lower back to take the strain.

Don't overwork your back for long periods. Take time to stretch regularly.

DIGGING
Digging can be hard work, especially if you have clay soil or are digging when the ground is wet. Sustained digging for a 30-minute period will burn an average of 120 calories.

THE ACTIVE GARDENING YEAR

Depending on where you live, gardening is a three-season or year-round occupation; there is always plenty to do to keep your garden in shape. The change of seasons is one of gardening's joys. It also makes the exercise that you get varied and interesting.

SPRING	SUMMER
Spiking lawn and raking out dead grass Repairing lawn with turf or sowing new seed Weeding Digging and raking seed beds Pruning and trimming hedges Dividing spring bulbs; planting summer bulbs Planting summer-flowering annuals Clipping hedges	Pruning spring-flowering shrubs Watering and deadheading bulbs and perennial flowers Spraying for insects and diseases Mowing lawns, trimming edges, and regularly removing clippings from lawn Planting and harvesting summer vegetables Planting root vegetables for autumn harvest Clipping hedges
AUTUMN	WINTER (SOUTHERN REGIONS)
Harvesting vegetables Clearing greenhouse and borders Clearing old crop and compost debris Digging and forking over the ground and adding compost Raking up leaves and clearing paths Planting winter vegetables	Clearing paths of weeds and moss Planting bare-root trees Digging out annuals Digging and forking over borders and adding manure and compost Raking seed beds Pruning fruit trees and shrubs

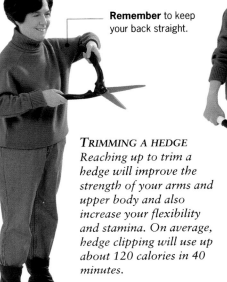
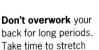

Origins

As a child, German Josef Pilates was plagued by asthma and rickets. Determined to improve his health, he studied different forms of exercise from both the East and the West. During the First World War, Pilates devised machines to help rehabilitate soldiers who were disabled by injury or disease. These were the prototypes of the Pilates equipment of today. In the 1920s Josef Pilates emigrated to America to set up an exercise studio. His exercises became popular with many ballet dancers of the time.

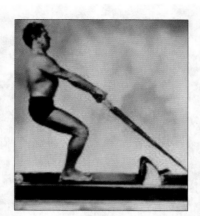

JOSEF PILATES (1880–1967)
The exercise system he devised more than 80 years ago has been used by countless people to improve strength, lose weight, and overcome injuries.

PILATES

Pilates is a system of gentle body stretches that are performed against pulleys or springs that provide resistance and prevent injury. The exercise system allows bone mass to be increased without the stress of gravity and also strengthens the muscles. Older people who have back problems, are recovering from strokes, or have had hip replacements can use the Pilates system to strengthen and realign their bodies.

The method is not used exclusively for rehabilitation, however; it has long been adopted by dancers and athletes to acquire strength without increasing muscle bulk. Pilates exercises, which require intense concentration, stretch and strengthen every part of the body. This is beneficial for people of every age but especially for anyone older than 50, for whom maintaining balance and flexibility is of prime importance. Teachers of the Pilates system describe it as a slow process of changing body habits and eliminating structural problems. It can be an excellent basis for gaining control over the care and health of the body.

WEIGHT AND APPETITE

Regular exercise increases metabolism, the rate at which you burn energy. Your basal metabolic rate (BMR) is a measure of your health and fitness. It is measured by calculating how much energy you use when you are inactive—such as while sleeping or lying down. Muscles burn more energy than fat; therefore, as you exercise and increase your muscle mass, you will also increase your BMR. This allows you to enjoy food without putting on weight. It is particularly important to maintain a healthy and stable weight to decrease the risk of heart disease, hypertension, high cholesterol, diabetes, gallstones, and arthritis.

Maintaining a healthy intake of nutrients is just as important as avoiding obesity. If you find yourself losing weight or the desire for food as you grow older, exercise can stimulate your appetite. This will help you stay at a healthy weight.

Boosting your metabolism and appetite will also increase your energy levels, helping you to overcome lethargy or apathy and even to fight depression.

Although you may feel tired when first embarking on a new exercise program, in only a few weeks you will notice the positive effects and begin to feel fitter. You will find your energy levels boosted and will sleep more soundly. Don't exercise just before going to bed, however, as it will probably make you too alert. Regular exercise will also help to soothe general aches and pains, provided you have no underlying injuries or conditions.

WHY YOU SHOULD GET ACTIVE NOW

Insufficient exercise at any age will lead to deterioration of the body. These include

▶ *An increase in the proportion of fat to muscle in your body*

▶ *Less efficient use of oxygen by the body*

▶ *Less efficient heart function—it pumps less blood per beat and has to work harder to get blood around the body*

▶ *A diminished sense of balance*

▶ *Impairment of the ability to control your body's internal temperature*

▶ *Fewer red blood cells and an increased tendency to form blood clots*

▶ *An increase in total blood fats, including cholesterol, which can cause problems*

▶ *Loss of calcium from bones*

▶ *Insensitivity to glucose in the blood, which increases the risk of diabetes*

EXERCISE FOR PEOPLE OVER 50

Exercise in your later years can improve your strength and flexibility; increase your metabolism; improve insulin sensitivity, appetite, and breathing; and help you remain independent.

Beginning or maintaining an exercise program should not cause you to change your life dramatically. As with all endeavors, making extreme changes seldom succeeds. You are more likely to adopt an effective and enjoyable exercise regimen by making simple adaptations to your lifestyle. This will reduce your chances of quitting should your other commitments increase. It is easy to find excuses for not exercising—being too busy, for example.

However, exercise will increase the energy you have for other tasks. It is well worth the effort of including an activity session in your daily routine.

Dispelling negative attitudes

The increasing availability of health clubs has prompted many people to join. But some persons may feel intimidated by seemingly complicated weight machines and by the image frequently attached to gyms.

EXERCISE MADE EASY

Exercise is involved in many daily tasks—climbing stairs, vacuuming, ironing, gardening, and carrying shopping bags, for example. The traditional concept of having exercise becomes much more accessible if

you grasp this perception of it. You don't have to join a gym in order to get fit—your daily tasks will provide plenty of scope for exercise—and every exercise effort will help toward your fitness goal.

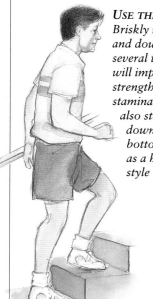

USE THE STAIRS
Briskly walking up and down stairs several times a day will improve your strength and stamina. You could also step up and down using the bottom two steps as a home step-style workout.

WALK TO THE STORE
Walk to the store or to social gatherings instead of using a car or bus. A lightweight shopping cart is a convenient and safe way to carry groceries or other purchases home.

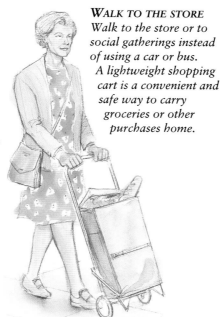

GET AN EXERCISE BIKE
If you invest in home equipment, such as weights or an exercise machine, then why not read a book, listen to music, or watch a video or television while you are exercising? Make the activity as enjoyable as possible.

EXERCISE AT A LOW COST

With a few simple measures you can keep fit without spending vast amounts of money.

▸ *Walk often; except for what you spend on shoes, it is free.*

▸ *For weight training, use filled water bottles or cans of food or buy elastic resistance bands.*

▸ *Take exercise classes at a community center. The fees are usually minimal.*

▸ *Find out if any gyms or health clubs in your area offer reduced rates for seniors.*

▸ *Buy only essential exercise gear, such as shoes, sports bra or jock strap, goggles, helmet.*

Older people especially may be intimidated because gyms and health clubs seem to be frequented by many of the young and fit.

Some exercises and sports have been perceived as competitive activities, which may generate a reluctance in some people to participate. Exercise, however, is an individual choice and should be chosen to suit your own needs. There are many ways to exercise—alone, with a friend, or in a more competitive environment if you choose.

Personal goals are crucial for adherence to an exercise program, and no matter what your goals are—whether they are to lose weight, become fit, improve your appearance, or prepare for a holiday—they are reason enough because a healthy lifestyle is always productive.

DIFFERENT TYPES OF EXERCISE

There are three components of physical fitness: endurance (stamina), muscular strength, and flexibility. All of these are equally important for preventing the detrimental effects of aging and for maintaining good overall health.

Aerobic exercise for stamina

Aerobic exercise should last for at least 12 minutes at a time and increase the heart rate. This type of exercise uses oxygen to provide energy for the muscles. Aerobic exercise of at least moderate intensity is the most effective way to improve the efficiency of your heart and lungs and to burn off fat.

If you have a sedentary lifestyle or if you are new to exercise, you should start with a less intense activity, such as walking. As your fitness improves, you can increase both the intensity and the duration until you are exercising for at least 20 minutes three times a week at a level that increases your heart

FUEL FOR EXERCISE

Exercise improves your appetite, so it is important to eat healthful foods rather than sweets and fat-laden snacks. Eat plenty of whole-grain bread, rice, and cereal, as well as fruits and vegetables. These will provide a ready supply of energy and the nutrients you need to stay healthy.

EXERCISE AND BODY TEMPERATURE

As you age, your ability to control your body temperature declines because of a lower metabolic rate and decreased ability to shiver (which generates heat). Also, because the heart does not pump as much blood per beat, there is decreased blood flow to the skin, and heat cannot escape from the body as quickly as it needs to. Exercise can improve the body's temperature control mechanism by

▸ *Increasing the amount of water in your body*

▸ *Increasing the amount you sweat; fit people also have more diluted sweat and thus lose fewer vitamins and minerals*

▸ *Improving cardiac output (the amount of blood the heart pumps) so that heat can be lost through the skin more efficiently*

▸ *Stimulating metabolism*

rate to 70 percent of maximum. Regular aerobic exercise is the only way to improve stamina. Good aerobic exercise includes any activity that raises your heartbeat and leaves you slightly out of breath, such as a brisk walk, an energetic swim, or a dance class.

Exercise for strength

Exercise that involves lifting weights or doing some other resistance training, such as push-ups, will improve muscle and bone strength. However, if you participate in strength training programs three times a week, you should also increase the amount of calories you consume. This is because muscle tissue requires more energy, or calories, to sustain its function. Therefore, as your muscles grow in size and strength, so will your need for calories.

Aim for moderate-intensity resistance training twice weekly. This involves approximately 8 to 10 exercises that work the main muscle groups, repeating them between 8 and 12 times (see pages 110–111). The main muscle groups are in the legs and pelvic area, the back and shoulders, the arms and chest, and the torso. Older adults benefit most from working muscles in the lower body because this can improve mobility and prevent falls. Toning or body-conditioning classes that require such equipment as light handheld weights or elastic training bands can also be effective for improving and maintaining strength. Less direct strength gains can be achieved from the aerobic activities mentioned above.

Older adults take longer physiologically to adapt to training programs and should aim to build strength gradually. If you are using free weights, always use them under supervision because there is a risk of overstraining muscles. The gym is the safest environment in which to learn about weight training and the equipment involved. There a qualified instructor can devise a strength training regimen specific to your age and ability. The program can then be adjusted as your ability increases.

Exercise for flexibility

Training for flexibility by performing stretches improves balance and agility, which are of utmost importance to elderly people. This sort of exercise also reduces muscular tension, improves posture and coordination, and enhances the ability to relax because stiffness is reduced.

Stretching exercises should never involve bouncing or jerking movements. In order to stretch the muscle and to effect a significant improvement in flexibility, a stretch should be executed slowly and held in one position for at least 15 to 45 seconds.

You should practice stretches at least three times a week. There are various ways you can incorporate them into your exercise routine. Most formal gym classes include some stretching, but you can also attend classes designed specifically for stretching.

BEFORE YOU BEGIN

Before embarking on any new exercise program, always consult your doctor. This is important not only to find out if you are fit enough to do the exercise but also to make sure that any underlying problems are identified and your family medical history is documented. Your doctor should check your weight and blood pressure and see if you have any joint, bone, cardiovascular, or respiratory problems.

Checking your pulse

The resting pulse is regarded by most experts as the best measure of fitness level, and it is certainly the easiest test you can perform. You can find your pulse in the radial artery of the inner wrist or in the carotid artery, which is found by following an imaginary line from the outer corner of your eye to your neck. In either case, use only your fingers (not your thumb) to locate your pulse. The average pulse rate for a woman is 78 to 84 beats per minute (bpm) and for men it is 72 to 78, although this range rises slightly with age.

The target training zone is the range in which you can intensify your level of exercise safely. This zone lies between 55 and 85 percent of your maximum heart rate, which is calculated by subtracting your age from 220 (see the box below). If you are a new exerciser, you should train at the lower end of the zone. As you become fitter, train toward the upper end. A simple way to monitor your exertion during exercise is the talk test: if you are unable to talk at all while working out, you are exercising too hard and should slow down.

Take your pulse 5 minutes after you have finished exercising to check your recovery heart rate; it should not exceed 60 percent of your personal maximum. For example, in a 50-year-old with a maximum heart rate of 170, this would be 102 bpm. The recovery heart rate is another indication of an individual's fitness levels; that is, the fitter the individual, the faster the pulse recovers.

TARGET TRAINING ZONE

Your optimum level of exercise can be estimated by calculating what is known as the target training zone, which is worked out from your maximum safe heart rate. Your maximum heart rate is equal to 220 minus your age. Your target training zone is between 55 and 85 percent of this maximum rate.

AGE	MAX HEART RATE (BPM)	TARGET (BPM)
50	170	94–145
55	165	91–140
60	160	88–136
65	155	85–131
70	150	83–128
75	145	80–123
80	140	77–119

Taking your pulse
You can take your pulse either in your neck or on your wrist. Don't use your thumb because it has a separate pulse of its own.

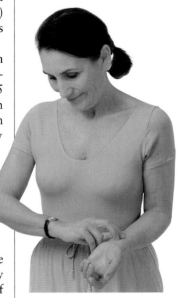

MEASURING YOUR PULSE
To measure the pulse in your wrist, press on the thumb side of your arm about 5 cm (2 in) above your wrist crease to find your radial artery. Count the beats for 15 seconds and then multiply by 4 to determine the beats per minute.

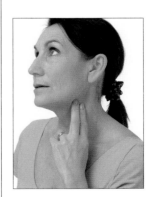

CAROTID ARTERY
Find the pulse in your neck by following an imaginary line from the outer corner of your eye to your neck.

Warm-up and Flexibility

The program illustrated over the next six pages provides a starting point for improving your stamina, strength, and flexibility. The exercises below and opposite are a basic warm-up routine combined with stretches to limber the body.

GENERAL WARMING UP TO LOOSEN MUSCLES

The purpose of a warm-up session is to prepare the body for exercise and reduce the risk of injury. It should last a minimum of 8 to 10 minutes and include all the major muscle groups. Walking is a gentle form of warming up that will improve blood flow and warm your muscles in preparation for stretching; this is vital in order to avoid muscle strain.

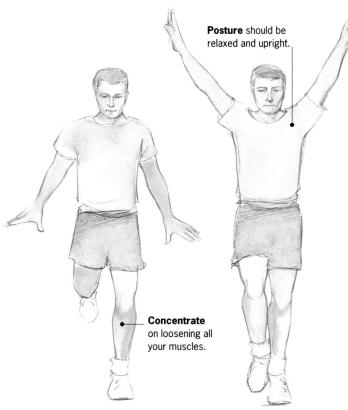

Concentrate on loosening all your muscles.

Posture should be relaxed and upright.

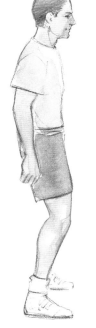

Breathing should be regular throughout the exercises.

1 *Begin by walking briskly. As you walk, circle your wrists, open and close your hands, rotate your shoulders, and squeeze your shoulders up and down.*

2 *Continue walking. Breathe in and stretch your arms upward in a circular motion; exhale and bring them down again. Your walking warm-up should last for at least 8 minutes.*

3 *End your warm-up by standing with your feet shoulder width apart, knees slightly bent, and stomach pulled in. Pull your stomach in further so your pelvis tilts forward. Hold for a slow count of eight. Uncurl and repeat.*

AVOIDING INJURY

▶ Always warm up prior to exercise and cool down afterward.

▶ Wear appropriate clothing. Too much is better than too little to maintain warmth. You can shed excess layers when necessary.

▶ Use appropriate gear and keep it well maintained; the correct footwear for walking will not be suitable for running.

▶ Remember to eat 1½ to 2 hours before exercising to provide energy and avoid cramping.

▶ Rehydrate regularly. Exercise will increase your need for fluid.

▶ "No pain, no gain" is an outdated concept. Exercise should not leave you exhausted, uncomfortable, in pain, or gasping for breath.

▶ Take your pulse regularly to make sure you stay within your target training zone (see page 105).

▶ If your goal is weight loss, aim to lose a maximum of ½ to 1 kg (1 to 2 lb) a week. Too rapid weight loss is not likely to be permanent and is a potential health risk.

▶ If you feel unwell or are recuperating from an illness, check with your doctor before restarting your exercise program.

▶ Exercise slowly and precisely, with no sudden movements.

STRETCHES FOR YOUR ARMS AND LEGS

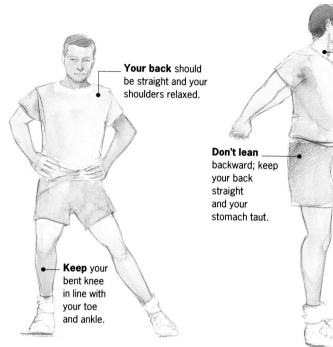

Your back should be straight and your shoulders relaxed.

Your neck should not jut forward.

Don't lean backward; keep your back straight and your stomach taut.

Keep your bent knee in line with your toe and ankle.

4 *Bend your right leg, keeping your knee in line with your foot and ankle, to gently stretch your left thigh. Hold for a count of eight. Repeat with the other leg.*

5 *Stand with your back straight, hands clasped behind your back. Lift your ribs to stretch the pectoral muscles across the chest. Hold for a count of eight.*

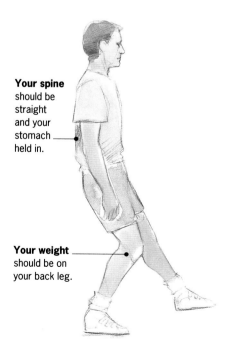

Your spine should be straight and your stomach held in.

Your weight should be on your back leg.

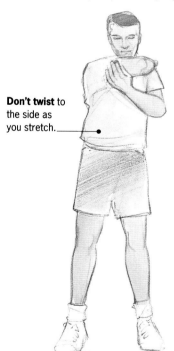

Don't twist to the side as you stretch.

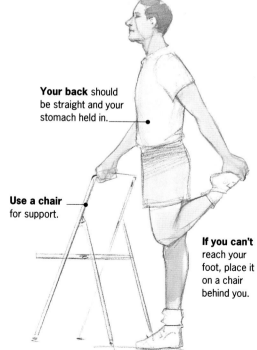

Your back should be straight and your stomach held in.

Use a chair for support.

If you can't reach your foot, place it on a chair behind you.

6 *Bend both legs and extend one in front of you on the floor. Hold for a count of eight; repeat on the other side.*

7 *Hold your shoulder with the opposite arm. Gently push it with your hand for a count of eight, then change sides.*

8 *Lift your left foot behind you and hold it with your left hand for a count of eight; repeat with the other leg.*

Aqua Aerobics

Aerobic exercise is vital for basic fitness. By exercising in the water, you can get the benefits of stamina and strength-building exercises without straining your joints and muscles. This is particularly helpful for people recovering from injuries.

POOLSIDE STRETCHES FOR THE BACK AND LEGS

WARMING UP

As with any other form of exercise, it is important to warm yourself up before you start. Either perform the warm-up exercises described on pages 106–107 or swim a couple of lengths, starting off gently and gradually increasing your speed. Alternatively, wade through the water for a couple of pool widths. After your aqua aerobics session, swim for a few minutes, gradually decreasing your pace. This will cool you down and prevent your muscles from aching.

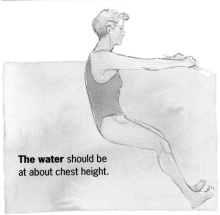

The water should be at about chest height.

1 *Face the side of the pool and place your feet low on the pool wall, with your knees bent.*

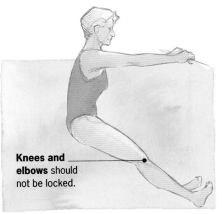

Knees and elbows should not be locked.

2 *Straighten your legs while keeping your hips level and your back straight. Hold for 8 to 10 seconds.*

UPPER BODY TONE-UP TO STRENGTHEN ARMS AND SHOULDERS

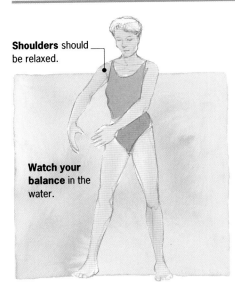

Shoulders should be relaxed.

Watch your balance in the water.

1 *Stand with your feet fairly wide apart and extend your arms out in front of you. Cup your hands as if you were holding a ball.*

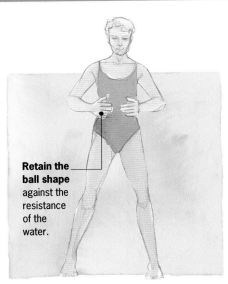

Retain the ball shape against the resistance of the water.

2 *Swing your hands in a figure-eight pattern through the water. Keep your shoulders level and your hands in the ball position throughout.*

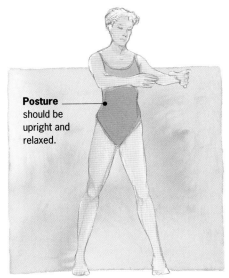

Posture should be upright and relaxed.

3 *Repeat the figure-eight movement 10 times. You will feel the resistance of the water working your arm and shoulder muscles.*

WATER MARCHING TO IMPROVE STAMINA

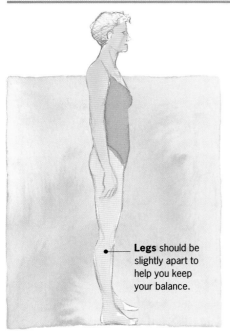

Legs should be slightly apart to help you keep your balance.

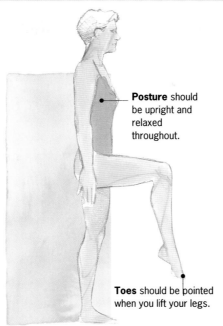

Posture should be upright and relaxed throughout.

Toes should be pointed when you lift your legs.

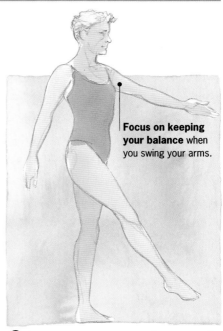

Focus on keeping your balance when you swing your arms.

1 *Stand up straight with your legs slightly apart and begin marching in place, lifting your knees up high. Concentrate on keeping your balance.*

2 *Resistance from the water keeps you moving in slow motion and makes your muscles work harder. Stretch your limbs as you march and point your toes.*

3 *Swing your arms to produce a good rhythmic walking movement. Aim to walk for at least 2 minutes or until you feel slightly breathless.*

WATER JUMPS TO INCREASE HEART RATE

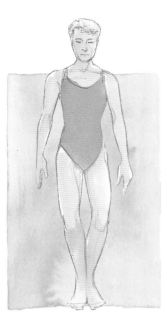

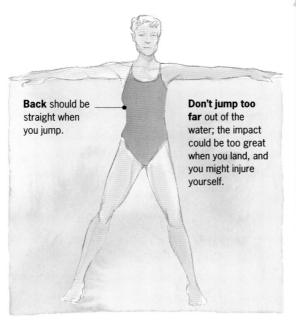

Back should be straight when you jump.

Don't jump too far out of the water; the impact could be too great when you land, and you might injure yourself.

1 *Stand straight with your arms relaxed by your sides. Bend your knees and spring upward but don't try to jump too high.*

2 *As you jump, kick your legs out and raise your arms to shoulder level. Make sure you keep your back straight and stomach pulled in. If you have any joint problems, wear a buoyancy belt to lessen the impact (see right).*

POOL SAFETY

Exercising in water can be safe and rewarding for people with joint pains or injuries. However, the following precautions should be taken to prevent injury.

▶ Make all movements gently and never lock your knees and elbows or jump too far out of the water.

▶ Tell the instructor about any specific health problems that you suffer from.

▶ Wear a buoyancy belt to reduce stress on your joints, especially if you have arthritis.

BUOYANCY BELT
A buoyancy belt decreases resistance and helps you keep your balance in the water.

Strength Exercises

The goal in strength training is to achieve balanced muscle strength; exercising only one group of muscles may cause weaknesses to develop elsewhere. However, strengthening the lower body in particular may greatly improve your mobility.

STANDING PRESS TO TONE ARMS AND SHOULDERS

The exercises below form a complete strength training program. If some muscles are already well developed, you can correct any imbalance by concentrating on the neglected muscle groups. As you get stronger, slowly increase the number of repetitions in each exercise.

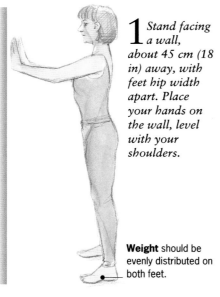

1 *Stand facing a wall, about 45 cm (18 in) away, with feet hip width apart. Place your hands on the wall, level with your shoulders.*

Weight should be evenly distributed on both feet.

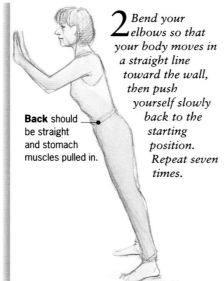

2 *Bend your elbows so that your body moves in a straight line toward the wall, then push yourself slowly back to the starting position. Repeat seven times.*

Back should be straight and stomach muscles pulled in.

ADDUCTOR TONER TO STRENGTHEN LEGS AND STOMACH

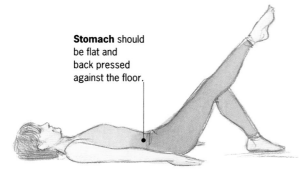

Stomach should be flat and back pressed against the floor.

1 *Lie on your back and bend both knees so that your feet are flat on the floor. Extend one leg in front of you, keeping your knees parallel.*

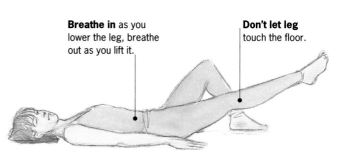

Breathe in as you lower the leg, breathe out as you lift it.

Don't let leg touch the floor.

2 *Slowly lower the leg toward the floor. Lift the leg to knee level again. Repeat seven more times to make a set, then change sides.*

SQUAT PLIÉ TO TONE HIPS, THIGHS, AND HAMSTRINGS

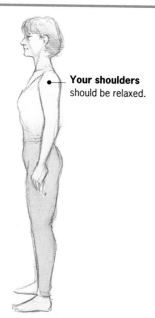

Your shoulders should be relaxed.

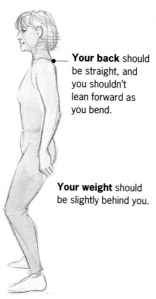

Your back should be straight, and you shouldn't lean forward as you bend.

Your weight should be slightly behind you.

1 *Stand with your feet about shoulder width apart, knees slightly bent, abdominals in, and back in alignment.*

2 *Breathe in and lower your body 5 cm (2 in) as if to sit down. Hold for a slow count of eight and return to the start position while breathing out. Repeat about seven times.*

AFTER EXERCISING

Aromatherapy can help relax your muscles and soothe any aches and pains after an exercise session. To make a soothing massage oil, add 4 drops of marjoram oil, 6 drops of eucalyptus oil, and 5 drops of rosemary oil to 50 ml (3 tbsp) of a base oil. Alternatively, try soaking in a warm bath to which 2 drops each of rosemary, eucalyptus, and lavender oils have been added.

Homeopathy may help relieve both muscle aches and joint pain. Arnica can help soothe painful muscles, while Bryonia may benefit stiff, swollen joints that are more painful after movement and exposure to heat. Nux vomica can relieve joint pain in which the symptoms are more painful when it is cold.

FLOOR EXERCISES TO FLATTEN STOMACH AND STRENGTHEN INNER THIGHS

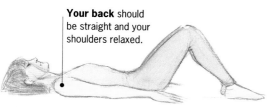

Your back should be straight and your shoulders relaxed.

1 *Lie on your back with both knees bent and your feet flat on the floor.*

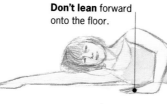

Don't lean forward onto the floor.

1 *Turn onto your side with your legs stretched out, one on top of the other. Rest your head on your arm.*

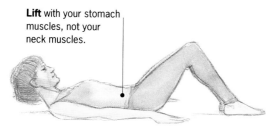

Lift with your stomach muscles, not your neck muscles.

2 *Breathe in, then as you breathe out, lift your head and raise your shoulders about 1 cm (½ in) and tighten your abdominals. Repeat the whole process 10 times.*

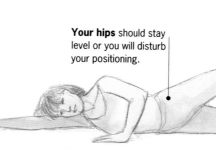

Your hips should stay level or you will disturb your positioning.

2 *As you breathe out, lift your top leg at least 5 cm (2 in) upward. As you breathe in, lower your leg but do not relax. Repeat slowly eight times. Repeat with the other leg.*

OVERCOMING MOBILITY PROBLEMS

Many older people may be wary of exercising because they have problems with mobility, but every individual should be able to find some form of exercise suitable for his or her needs.

Many older people suffer from stiff joints, arthritis, or general aches that can make beginning an exercise program difficult. While no one should ever exercise to the point where it causes great pain, there are ways of lessening the pain experience and adapting popular exercises to suit particular abilities.

If you suffer from joint difficulties, once you begin to exercise regularly, you will probably find your pain levels lessening over time. Exercise improves flexibility and lubricates joints, thus reducing stiffness. If you exercise for more than 20 minutes (which may not be possible at first), the exercise will prompt your brain to release natural painkilling chemicals known as endorphins.

Even if the only activity you can manage is to walk a short distance, you should persevere. You will soon be able to do more. Before beginning, however, see your doctor to discuss exercise options. If you have specific difficulties, a doctor can refer you to a physiotherapist or osteopath, who may be able to extend your range of movement by a

MIND OVER MATTER

Two American studies have shown that making positive statements during a painful experience, either silently to yourself or out loud, can help to reduce pain. Researchers E. Fernandez in 1986 and Delia Cioffi and James Holloway in 1993 found that making a statement such as "The pain is uncomfortable but not unbearable" or "This hurts, but I'm still in control and okay" helped people to cope better with pain.

combination of heat treatment, manipulation, and gentle exercise. There are other alternative forms of treatment that can also relieve pain, allowing you to exercise without resorting to drugs that may become addictive and ineffective over time. For example, with TENS (transcutaneous nerve stimulation), two small pads are attached to the skin over or beside the painful area, and a small battery-operated unit passes a mild electric current between the pads. The level of the current's intensity is controlled by the person experiencing the pain. The current masks the pain by stimulating the nerves below the skin's surface.

If you suffer from chronic pain, it may be worthwhile trying relaxation therapies as a means of overcoming the problem. Much recent research has focused on the role of stress in increasing our perception of pain. Expecting to experience pain when you place weight on a joint or exercise vigorously may be enough to cause muscle tension, anxiety, and fear—all of which will heighten feelings of pain. Therapies such as meditation and creative visualization can help you overcome any such expectations of pain, while a relaxing massage or aromatherapy session before attempting exercise may help relax your muscles and make them more receptive to exercise.

Many people find that a session of autogenic training is very effective in helping to overcome the negative expectation of pain. The technique, based on the work of neuropsychiatrist Johannes Schultz, has been practiced for more than 50 years. Autogenic training teaches you to trigger your parasympathetic nervous system (the part of the nervous system that is not under your voluntary control) and promotes relaxation and rest. The method is usually taught by

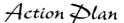

CASE STUDY

A Retired Exerciser

After retiring many people find themselves becoming more sedentary. Being physically inactive increases the risk of many conditions associated with aging, such as stiff joints and osteoporosis. It may also prevent people from living as full a life as possible. There are numerous benefits, both physical and mental, from taking up exercise after retirement.

Val, aged 62, retired two years ago from her job as a high school English teacher. Her working day typically involved a lot of standing, walking, and carrying heavy books around. Despite still having good physical stamina and being a healthy weight for her height, Val feels increasingly tired and stiff. During the day she takes care of her grandchildren, a three-year-old and a nine-month-old, while her daughter goes to work. Val often suffers from backache and finds it frustrating that she can't keep up with the older child as well as she would like to. Sometimes she finds it difficult to pick up the baby, and she worries about caring for the children properly. Val would like to strengthen her back with exercise.

WHAT SHOULD VAL DO?

Val should first see her doctor for a checkup to make sure her backache is not a sign of something serious. Once given the go-ahead, she should look for some gentle exercise that suits her needs and that will not overly stress her back.

Her friend Alice already attends a yoga class, so Val could go along with her to a session to see if she would enjoy it. By explaining her particular level of fitness and her health concerns to the teacher and starting the class at her own pace, she would minimize any initial pain. Also, practicing the exercises at home would improve her flexibility more rapidly. She may also need to rethink how she manages the children.

Action Plan

EXERCISE
Find an exercise class at an appropriate level and discuss aims with the teacher. Practice stretches slowly and carefully.

LIFESTYLE
Attend a yoga class at least twice a week to keep up new levels of strength and suppleness.

FAMILY
Be careful not to overreach and injure stiff muscles while looking after children. Have a stretching session during the day; invite the older child to join in for fun.

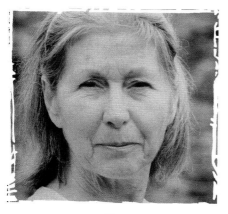

FAMILY
Family commitments can be hard to meet if you are experiencing pain.

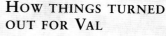

EXERCISE
Any new exercise program must be undertaken gradually, and great care should be taken to prevent injury.

LIFESTYLE
Limited mobility from lack of exercise can compromise the ability to carry out everyday tasks and responsibilities.

HOW THINGS TURNED OUT FOR VAL

After checking with her doctor, Val joined Alice in the yoga class. She thoroughly enjoyed herself and began attending twice a week, as well as practicing at home. She found the stretches fun, and the breathing exercises and meditation helped her relax after a hectic day with the children. Val found herself becoming stronger and more supple. As an unexpected bonus, her posture improved and she had far more energy.

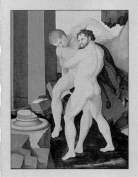

The Labors of Hercules
Even in Greek mythology exercise and physical labor were connected to longevity or immortality. Hercules was given the task of performing 12 impossibly arduous feats in order to become immortal, and in the process he developed great physical strength and prowess. Eventually he was rewarded by being accepted among the gods.

SWIMMING CHAMPIONS
In 1995 the men's world record for 50-meter freestyle swimming in the 55–59 age group was 27.05 seconds. The world record for the same distance in the 80–84 age group was 34 seconds. The difference in time between the two groups is surprisingly small, showing that if you are fit, age need not slow you down.

doctors, nurses, or psychologists and relies on "passive concentration." You are led through routines, such as making your arm feel heavy, until you reach a deep state of concentration. Some people have found autogenic training so effective that they no longer depend so heavily on medications such as painkillers or tranquilizers.

HEALTH CLUBS

Health clubs can be very beneficial to older people who have mobility problems because such facilities contain a range of equipment that can specifically target areas of the body where strength needs to be increased or mobility restored. Designing a program with a physiotherapist or a gym instructor will help you choose machinery that eases the weight load on a particular joint or works a weak muscle without excessive strain. Many health clubs also offer a range of other facilities, such as a sauna, swimming pool, and massage room, any of which can help you prepare stiff or painful muscles and joints for exercise and to recover from a strenuous session.

A good health club should give you a full fitness assessment when you join to determine an appropriate exercise program for you, and you should receive full training on all resistance and cardiovascular machines.

SPORTS

It can be very dispiriting to find you can no longer take part in a favorite sport because of injury or ill health. However, many people give up on sports long before they need to. With a few simple adaptations, most sports can be made accessible and less of a

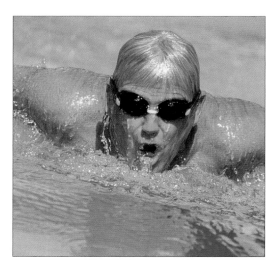

strain. Keeping up with an enjoyable form of exercise is more likely to help in any recovery process rather than hinder it.

Cycling

According to the British Medical Association, cycling 8 km (5 miles) four times a week halves your risk of heart disease. Cycling is a low-impact activity, so it is ideal for people with joint problems. Older people should avoid bicycling on busy roads, however, because the sense of balance can become impaired with age. Cycling in parks and on quiet country roads may be more suitable. Most bicycles are easy to transport on an automobile bicycle rack. Some have front wheels that can be removed or frames that can be folded up so you don't even need a rack. Consider also buying an exercise bike for indoors or convert your old bicycle to a stationary model. Remember, you don't have to use an exercise bike indoors. If you miss being out in the open air, move your bike to the garden and pedal there.

Walking

Walking is probably the ideal low-impact, low-risk, and low-cost activity. It is a good measure of mobility and therefore is the form of exercise that is most beneficial to develop. You may be anxious about walking alone as you grow older, particularly if you have mobility problems that slow you down and make you feel more vulnerable. If this is the case, the ideal way to keep walking is to invite a friend to accompany you or join a walking club. Many clubs are aimed specifically at older people, so it possible to find one with an intensity level that suits your needs. You could also investigate historic or scenic walks in your area. In addition to being good exercise, these walks are often very stimulating, and many incorporate stops in cafés for rest breaks.

Squash and tennis

Many doctors discourage people over the age of 50 from taking up squash because the sudden bursts of activity characteristic of the game can cause injury or even a heart attack (if a blood clot is dislodged). Tennis, on the other hand, can be played at much lower intensities and, particularly if you play doubles, places far less strain and physical demand on you, yet the sport will still keep you active and fit. The benefits of the

Getting Fit with

Line Dancing

People of any age and fitness level can enjoy line dancing. A country dance that originated in America's southwestern states, line dancing is fun for people of all ages, and it has become popular all over North America and Europe.

If you are a fan of country and western music, then you might find line dancing a very enjoyable form of exercise. It is an excellent way to maintain fitness and give your social life a boost at the same time. If you are single, it is not daunting because you do not need a partner to take

part. Because line dancing is mostly step work, it is unlikely to put strain on your back or other parts of your body, and it carries a low risk of injury. It is not overly strenuous and is suitable for people who are unfit or need to take things slowly because of an injury.

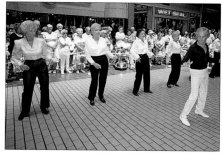

DANCE CRAZE
Line dancing has long been an important part of social events in the United States; exhibitions by line dance groups are common events throughout the country.

A STEP-BY-STEP LINE DANCE

This simple routine is known as a vine dance and is very popular with beginners. It demonstrates how easy it is to participate in line dancing and is excellent as a warm-up before attempting the more demanding dance routines. This dance also helps

beginners to become familiar with dancing in a line. A line dance session has a physical effect on the body similar to that of a low-impact aerobics class, making it a good cardiovascular exercise and beneficial to balance as well. It also helps

you maintain muscle tone and good posture, strength, and coordination. Dance the routine to any music with a regular 4/4 beat and make each movement on the beat. Repeat the sequence three more times until you are back at the start.

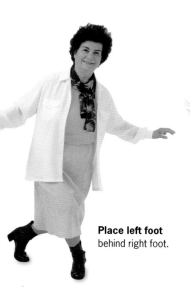

Place left foot behind right foot.

1 *Step your right foot to the right and swing your left leg behind it. Put your weight on your left foot and step to the right again. Lift your left leg up in front of you.*

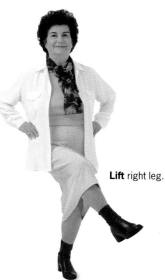

Lift right leg.

2 *Step your left foot to the left and then swing your right leg behind. Put your weight on your right foot and step to the left again. Lift your right leg up in front.*

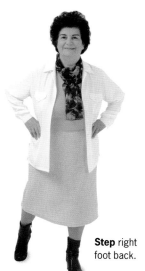

Step right foot back.

3 *Step your right foot back, then move your left leg back to meet it. Step your right foot back once more and then lift your left leg up in front of you.*

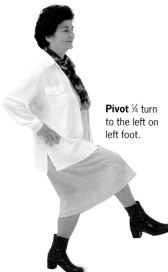

Pivot ¼ turn to the left on left foot.

4 *Step your left foot forward, then slide the right foot next to it. Step your left foot forward and lift up your right leg in front. Pivot ¼ turn on your left leg.*

115

Easing tendinitis
Inflammation of the tendons, known as tendinitis, can occur after too much exercise or exercising incorrectly. Try applying arnica cream to the affected area or soak a pad in a diluted tincture of the herb and apply it as a compress.

social aspect of sports such as tennis, for which a partner is required, should also not be overlooked.

Swimming

Swimming is one of the few activities that improves stamina, strength, and flexibility simultaneously. It is impact-free and has been used traditionally for postoperative rehabilitation and physiotherapy. Swimming is excellent exercise for the obese and for those who have ongoing orthopedic and arthritic conditions because the body weight is entirely supported by the water and therefore not subject to gravitational forces. If you have lower back problems, vary your stroke so that your head and neck are not constantly thrown backward. Many pools offer lap swimming at off-peak times, special sessions for seniors, swimming lessons, and aqua aerobics classes.

ALTERNATIVE EXERCISE

Yoga, an ancient approach to health and well-being developed in India some 5,000 years ago, is an excellent exercise for people of all ages. Yoga is also a philosophy but you do not have to become involved in its philosophical aspects to enjoy and benefit from the practice.

Yoga improves balance, suppleness, breathing, and body control—benefits that become increasingly important as you age. Many people also find yoga beneficial because sessions generally end with deep relaxation. This soothes muscles and eases stress and tension.

Although many forms of yoga are taught in the West, the method most commonly practiced is hatha yoga, which combines gentle stretches, called asanas, with breath-

ing exercises, called pranayamas. The asanas work each part of the body in turn and concentrate on stretching the spine. It is thought that the asanas also help improve the digestive and nervous systems and release tension. If you are a beginner, it is essential to attend classes in which you can learn the positions properly. If you have any medical problems, check with a doctor before starting a class.

T'ai chi is an ancient martial art that has been practiced in China for centuries. It is nonconfrontational, relaxing, and enjoyable. The movements in t'ai chi resemble a slow dance; indeed, it has been described as poetry in motion. Its emphasis is on strength, stability, control of the body, and suppleness. It is therefore an excellent form of exercise for older people.

Correct posture and foot placement are of utmost importance in t'ai chi. Each set of movements involves transferring weight slowly and gracefully and gently twisting and balancing the body. If you are a beginner, it is essential to attend classes to learn the movements correctly. After you have mastered them, you can practice on your own—15 minutes a day is all you need.

Dancing is fun, sociable, and an excellent form of exercise. If you are worried about being able to remain motivated to stay with an exercise program, dance may be a good exercise for you. All forms of dance improve balance, coordination, and agility, and there are many to choose from, including ballroom, ballet, jazz, folk, tap, line dancing, even belly dancing and flamenco. Most dance classes start with a warm-up and then progress to more vigorous exercises. Some classes, such as ballroom, may have a free dance session during which you can change partners and join in or sit out as you wish. In this way you can go at your own pace and not push yourself too hard. As with other forms of exercise, you should make sure you are moving for at least 20 minutes and that your level of activity is sufficient to raise your heartbeat.

If you suffer from backache or problems with your posture, you might find that a course in the Alexander technique helps. The technique is a movement therapy rather than a form of exercise, but it can improve balance, coordination, and posture and may help to prepare your body for the demands of more vigorous exercise.

ACHIEVING BALANCE
Yoga can increase your mobility by improving your flexibility and balance. You may even find that with regular classes and practice, you are more supple than ever before.

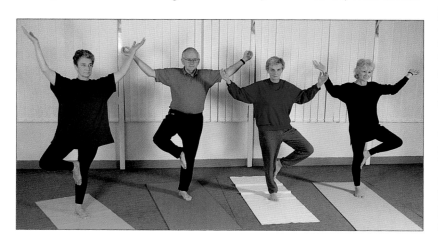

CHAPTER 6

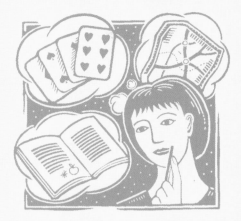

AN ACTIVE MIND

*Contrary to popular belief, the mind does
not deteriorate with age. You can promote good
brain function and strengthen your memory with a
variety of daily activities. Focusing on strategies to
help reduce the harmful effects of stress will also
help you maintain good mental balance.*

HOW AGING AFFECTS YOUR BRAIN

There is nothing inevitable about age-related mental decline. With proper stimulation and exercise our brains can remain alert and sharp well into old age.

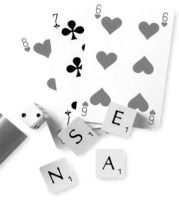

MIND GAMES
Games that involve memory, logic, or tactical thinking, such as cards or Scrabble, are excellent for keeping your mind alert and active.

Mental functions do not necessarily worsen as we age, but they do change. As the human mind ages, it loses some of its agility and quickness of response, just as the body does, but problem-solving skills and accuracy remain constant. Older people fare less well on conventional IQ tests because of the large number of categories—among them verbal, numerical, and abstract reasoning. But if the number of tests is reduced from the usual 11 to only 6, older people's performance equals that of young people in their prime.

The nervous system is capable of carrying messages at up to 426 km (265 miles) per hour when we are young. As we age, these top speeds fall by up to 15 percent. This change affects the rapidity but not the ability with which we tackle mental tasks. This was demonstrated by psychologist Neil Charness at the University of Waterloo in Ontario, Canada, who studied the performance of a group of bridge players. He found that there was no decrease in the accuracy of the bidding of older players, but they took longer to make their bids, a decline that worked out at roughly two-thirds of a second for every additional decade they had lived.

Some mental functions actually improve with age, particularly those that benefit from experience and learning. Dr. Elizabeth Maylor of the Medical Research Council's Applied Psychology Unit in Cambridge, England, provided evidence for this through her study of 100 contestants in *Mastermind*, a popular TV quiz show. She found that the older contenders were much more proficient on general knowledge than the younger ones. Their greater experience enabled them to make responses that were more accurate than those of their youthful rivals, and they made them more quickly.

Intelligence is not uniform over a range of skills, but different types of intelligence make an individual better at some activities than others. Two of these types are known as crystalized and fluid intelligence. Crystallized intelligence incorporates the knowledge acquired during a person's lifetime, whereas fluid intelligence is used to solve problems encountered in novel situations and draws very little upon acquired knowledge. Fluid intelligence seems to decline after the age of 50, but crystallized intelligence remains remarkably constant with age.

Older people also have the benefit of experience, which often enables them to act more decisively than those who are younger. Because of experience, older persons can be versatile in the way they achieve their aims, and they can get around declining abilities

A NEW LEASE ON LIFE

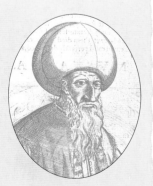

SINAN (1491–1588)
Late in life, Sinan created buildings that became monuments of an empire.

Sinan began work as an architect for Sultan Suleiman the Magnificent at the age of 47. Sinan's career lasted for 50 years, and he completed over 500 buildings, including palaces, hospitals, and magnificently ornate mosques. He was inspired by great Christian and pagan buildings, such as the Hagia Sophia in Istanbul and the Parthenon in Athens, and wished to re-create their grandeur in his own works. Sinan was in his eighties when he finished the Selimiye Mosque, regarded as one of the great buildings of the world.

by utilizing others. "Slow and steady wins the race" is usually the way older people reach their goals—frequently doing better at a task than younger, rasher, more impatient people.

THE BRAIN AND AGING

The brain, like the other muscles of the body, needs to be used regularly in order to maintain its ability to function well. The human adult brain contains approximately 100,000 million nerve cells (neurons), and every 10 years after about the age of 40 about 10 percent of these neurons die and are not replaced. As you age, connections between your neurons contract, widening the gap between them and thus slowing down your responses, coordination, reflexes, and reactions. However, you can help your brain to fend off these effects.

Neurons react to mental stimulation by creating new connections. These connections are made through extensions called axons and dendrites, the chemical messengers that carry information between cells. The longer axons connect nerve impulses to other neurons, and the shorter dendrites receive nerve impulses and send them to the cell body. These connections are considered especially important because they are the means by which brain cells interconnect with each other. Dendrites also decrease as people age. But research has shown that these, too, can be rejuvenated through stimulation of the mind.

Experiments on rats carried out at the University of California provided physiological evidence that the brain expands because of activity and stimulation. The researchers divided the rats into pairs. One pair was kept in an impoverished environment until their age was equivalent to the human age of 75 years (10 days in a rat's life is roughly equivalent to a year in a human life). The other pair was placed in an enriching environment. Subsequent anatomical studies revealed a far greater number of connections between the brain cells of the stimulated rats than those of the impoverished rats. The brain cells in the stimulated rats had also grown in size by 15 percent. Interestingly, in a further experiment rats that had been kept in an impoverished environment and then were transferred to an enriched one until their age was equivalent to a human age of 90 showed considerable growth in neural connections. The term coined to describe this sort of growth is structural plasticity.

Research has since been carried out to see whether the conclusions from the rat experiment can be applied to humans. In 1993 neuroscientist Bob Jacobs performed autopsies on elderly people, some of whom had been university graduates and some of whom had left school early. He found that those who were more highly educated had up to 40 percent more connections in their brains than the others. Although education can be seen as the human equivalent of the rats' enriched environment, Jacobs also discovered that those graduates who had continued to learn, to read, and to explore their environment had more brain connections

continued on page 122

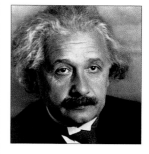

ALBERT EINSTEIN
An autopsy performed on Albert Einstein's brain showed a proliferation of the connecting fibers, or dendrites, 400 percent greater than in the average human brain.

STIMULATION AND THE BRAIN

Neurons in the brain are not joined to each other but are separated by a space called the synaptic gap. Each of these brain cells communicates with another by firing chemical messengers, or neurotransmitters, between the axons and the dendrites. If the brain is not regularly stimulated, the synaptic gap widens, making communication more difficult. Stimulation allows dendrites to proliferate and increases the ability to make connections between neurons. This helps compensate for the natural cell loss that occurs with aging.

THOUGHT PROCESS
Neurotransmitters reach their receptor points in other neurons over the synaptic gap. This allows more information to be processed.

axon

neuron

dendrite

axon terminal

neurotransmitters

synaptic gap

receptor site

The Neuro-Linguistic Programmer

Neuro-Linguistic Programming (NLP) is a way of closely observing your mind's processes and then adjusting them to create a more positive lifestyle and overcome obstacles or fears that may be preventing you from experiencing a full life.

OVERCOMING FEAR
Neuro-Linguistic Programming can be invaluable as a tool for overcoming stumbling blocks, such as a fear of public speaking. This could make events such as giving a speech much less stressful.

Origins

Neuro-Linguistic Programming began in California in the 1970s when mathematician Richard Bandler and linguist John Grinder set out to research what makes some people more successful than others. Taking inspiration from Gestalt therapy, pioneered by Fritz Perls, and three people who were experts in human behavior—Dr. Milton H. Erickson, a renowned hypnotherapist, Virginia Satir, a successful family therapist, and Gregory Bateson, an anthro-pologist—Bandler and Grinder observed minutely how these individuals worked, from the way they thought to how they moved and spoke. The scientists then recorded the exact processes that took place and the precise sequence in which they

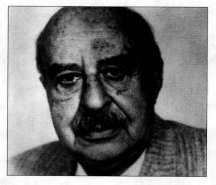

FRITZ PERLS
An outstanding psychotherapist, Perls developed therapeutic approaches that influenced the originators of NLP.

happened. From these findings they identified modes of thinking that seemed more likely to ensure excellence and success and created models to follow. The results evolved into Neuro-Linguistic Programming, which is now practiced around the world.

NLP is concerned with effective communication, whether it is with others or with yourself. The technique assumes that every event of the outside world is filtered by the senses, which in turn draw upon past experiences, making every person's view of life unique and subjective. Our minds form a map of the predictable thought processes that we go through when faced with an external experience. For example, if someone with a phobia of spiders comes across a picture of a spider in a magazine, he or she will react differently than someone who does not have such a fear. The outer experience is exactly the same, but the information is interpreted differently. NLP teaches people to manipulate these filters, or maps, in order to overcome negative or destructive thoughts and develop positive models for behavior.

How does NLP work?

NLP focuses on the practical ways to change unwanted behaviors. Research has indicated that language has a major effect on how people influence their own lives and communicate with themselves and others. NLP therefore concentrates on language and how experiences are labeled. People generally fall into one of three "patterns" of labeling: visual, auditory, or kinesthetic (feelings). Determining how you and others label your experiences enables you to change your perceptions or relate to others in a more constructive way.

What will a practitioner do?

During a session a practitioner will help you identify what you want to achieve, whether it is to become more confident socially, to be more assertive, or to overcome a particular fear. This process is perhaps harder than it sounds. Many people find it difficult to identify their goals or fears. A Neuro-Linguistic Programmer will help you clarify your aims by asking questions and then help you identify your habitual way of thinking by observing the language you use in your answers.

Communication through language is considered to be of key importance in relating to others and even to yourself effectively. For example, if you are a predominantly visual thinker, you might regularly use phrases like "I see what you mean" or "Let's take a look at this." People who are auditory are more likely to use such language as "I hear what you are saying," whereas those who think kinesthetically will "feel things in their bones."

Once you have identified your own habitual patterns, a practitioner will help you change unwanted ways of thinking and make your negative thoughts and fears more positive. With the help of the practitioner,

you can also use the technique to identify the mindsets of people who have been successful. You can then copy their methods and try to match their achievements. This technique is called modeling. For modeling to be successful, it is essential not only to understand the actions of the person who is being modeled but to investigate and understand that person's motivations and thought processes at the same time. This technique creates a map, or guide, in your own mind of how success can be achieved.

What type of problems can be addressed by NLP?

NLP can be applied to almost any task or goal because it is a way of training your mind. Initially, it was a study of excellence, investigating, for example, how one person finds it easy to learn languages but another is still not proficient after many years of study. NLP hoped to discover a method of learning that would enable everyone to achieve their full potential in any skill they wished.

Many athletes and businesspeople use the technique to motivate themselves, but NLP is applicable to retired people as well. During retirement it is sometimes necessary to confront situations that make you feel fearful or insecure—such as driving at night, dealing with money, or traveling alone. NLP can help you approach these things with a positive attitude. It is often very quick to take effect and can make tasks easier and more enjoyable to complete.

Evidence of the power of NLP is mounting. Studies suggest that NLP has even helped some people to overcome allergies by training the brain not to react to a potential allergen, thus influencing the immune system.

WHAT YOU CAN DO AT HOME

Begin by listing characteristics of yourself in one or two words, for example, self-confident, happy, shy, forgetful. Create your list using your nondominant hand (if you are right-handed, write with your left hand). When you use this method, your mind is able to reach a subconscious level and your list will be more honest. When you have finished, change to your dominant hand and expand each word into a more specific sentence. For example, if you have put down "shy," your sentence might be "I am too scared to talk to strangers."

Look at each of your sentences and try to establish the thought processes behind it. To do this, visualize one of your positive sentences, using all your senses to create a vivid picture of it in your mind. Then visualize one of your negative traits in the same way. Notice the differences in your thought patterns. If you apply your positive thought pattern to a negative scene, you are more likely to change your perception of events. As you practice this technique, you should be able to spot negative thoughts that you habitually use and change them for more positive ones.

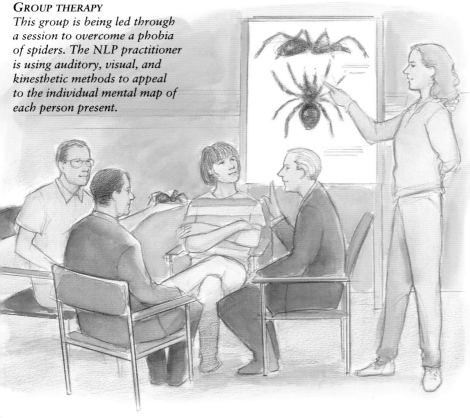

GROUP THERAPY
This group is being led through a session to overcome a phobia of spiders. The NLP practitioner is using auditory, visual, and kinesthetic methods to appeal to the individual mental map of each person present.

Music

According to some British research, brain rhythms can be affected by music. Three groups were asked to listen to three different pieces of music. The first group was given an excerpt from a piece by Mozart that was fast and fugal; the second listened to a slower-paced heavy rock piece, and the third group heard a soothing, slow, tranquil piece. The response patterns of the brain were stimulated and became more alert after listening to the quicker melodies of Mozart.

SURF THE NET
Getting acquainted with computers can give you easy access to a wide range of information via the Internet. Electronic mail can also help you stay in touch with family and friends more readily than regular mail.

than those who had become mentally sluggish in later life. This was the case whatever the original level of education the person had achieved.

There is no universal pattern for brain aging. Although we all lose cells and connections, making the most of what is left is what makes the difference. Up to the age of 70, it is reasonable to expect to retain most of your mental abilities, given the right stimulation. Often there is no change in learning ability, although the elderly are sometimes wrongly conditioned to believe that mental faculties become diminished with age.

MAINTAINING MENTAL FITNESS

Constant interaction with information that is unfamiliar forces the brain to exercise. It has to assess, question, and respond to new information being relayed and to assimilate it; therefore, being employed tends to lead to healthy brain functioning.

A survey of Japanese octogenarians concluded that individuals who continued to work a normal day in an office had greater mental agility than contemporaries who had retired at 60. There was greater mental agility even when the time spent in the office was just one hour a day.

Not everyone chooses or is able to continue working, but it is possible to find other ways to get daily mental stimulation to replace the stimulation of work following

retirement. For example, you can take on responsiblity in a community organization, social club, or political or nonprofit group. Ask questions, talk to people, find ways to become more involved. You could also think about ways of sharing your own knowledge with other people by tutoring. Meeting new people, conversing, and gaining new perspectives will all help to keep your mind active and stimulated.

Exercise and your brain

It is not just mental exercise that keeps your brain healthy. Physical activity also seems to be important. Researchers at the Institute of Ageing at Manchester University spent 12 years studying the brain function of a sample of 600 Britons aged 50 to 70. The research team found a correlation between fitness levels and retention of faculties. In the course of their investigations, they discovered that regular exercise helps to prevent mental decline. A physically fit 70-year-old can have the brain power of someone 20 years younger.

It seems that the fitter you are and the better you tolerate exercise, the easier it is for oxygen to reach the brain, as well as other organs and muscles. The exercise need not be vigorous to provide this improvement. Investigations carried out by Professor Gustav Holmann of Cologne University, Germany, have proved that even twiddling the fingers can improve blood flow to the brain by as much as one-quarter.

MEMORY AND AGING

A great concern of older people is the fear of losing their memory. However, memory loss is not a straightforward matter. There are at least three different types of memory: sensory, short-term, and long-term.

The process in which the sensory nerve cells in the brain learn to recognize patterns in the environment, such as letters of the alphabet is called sensory memory. This form of memory registers a great deal of information from the environment but holds it for only a very brief time (perhaps one-quarter of a second to three seconds). From this range of sensory information, your brain selects certain portions to be stored in short-term memory. Short-term, or working, memory holds all the information you are currently thinking about or are consciously aware of. It has a limited storage

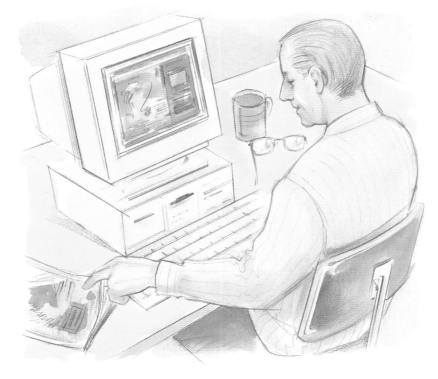

WHERE MEMORIES ARE STORED

The brain is such a complex and inaccessible organ that neuroscientists are a long way from completely understanding its mechanisms. However, through recent advances in brain research, they have been able to identify groups of cells, or neurons, that lie close to each other and connect easily. These cells seem to form a memory circuit. It was once thought that memories were stored throughout the brain, but recent research analyzing simple actions, such as blinking in response to light, in people suffering from brain injury or amnesia has revealed that different parts of the brain store different types of memories.

The amygdala is where memories associated with senses or emotions are stored, such as the knowledge that fire is hot.

INSIDE THE BRAIN
Different types of memories seem to be stored within different areas of the brain. This explains why someone suffering a disruption in brain function may be able to remember some things but not others.

The hippocampus is where new memories are formed and short-term memories are retained. It is here that most age-related changes occur.

The cerebellum is where memories associated with movement are stored, such as remembering how to ride a bicycle or how to walk.

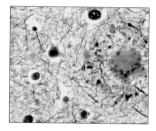

ALZHEIMER'S DISEASE
The dark area shown here is where neurons have degenerated into tangled clumps instead of ordered memory circuits, causing massive memory loss.

capacity—some research suggests we are able to store only seven items at a time—and storage is for a short period, perhaps only 30 seconds. Some items that are held briefly in short-term memory are then transferred to long-term memory, the form of memory that the majority of people are most aware of. It is where we store memories potentially for a lifetime.

Research and knowledge of the brain developed considerably during the 20th century. Experiments in which learned behavior was observed sought to establish precisely where in the brain different types of memory are stored. These were first carried out using subjects who were brain damaged or were suffering from amnesia. As technology improved, electrical sensors were used to detect activity in the brain. It appears that long-term, motor memories, such as how to walk, are stored in the back of the brain in an area called the cerebellum. Memories associated with the senses are stored in the amygdala at the front of the brain. Short-term memories are stored in the hippocampus. This is also the area where memories are apparently formed.

The ability to store recent events of no great importance in short-term memory declines with age. But long-term memory remains stable and can even become sharper. It is believed that the human brain can store 1,000 trillion items of information. However long we live, we are unlikely to fill this massive database. The memory lapse problem is not one of inadequate data storage but of imperfect information retrieval.

Even so, there is a great deal of misinformation about age-related memory impairment. Dr. Gene Cohen, acting director of the U.S. National Institute of Aging, found that changes once said to be related to aging may, in fact, be due to illness or even medication. An estimate made recently by a task force of American doctors suggests that 10 to 20 percent of people diagnosed with

OMEGA-3 FATTY ACIDS
Omega-3 fatty acids may contribute to healthy brain function. They help in the formation of neurotransmitters and cell membranes and also reduce "bad" cholesterol, which can restrict blood flow to the brain. Omega-3 fats are found in oily fish, nuts, polyunsaturated oils, and flaxseeds.

123

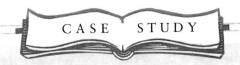

A Woman with Vitamin Deficiencies

Many people expect their brain function to deteriorate as they age. But these changes are not inevitable; our brains are capable of remaining sharp for our entire lives. Some cases of mental confusion or illness can be provoked, however, by general malnutrition or more specific nutrient deficiencies, which can easily be reversed and further prevented by attention to diet.

May is in her eighties and has lived on her own since the death of her housekeeper a year ago. She has been eating only sporadically but does drink a few glasses of wine every evening. Until recently she pursued an academic career and was still contributing to journals. Her family has become very concerned because lately May is confused and forgetful, has great difficulty walking, and is often short of breath. They took her to the family doctor, whom she has known for 40 years, and May was unable to recognize him. Because May's deterioration was so rapid, he advised the family to hospitalize her for tests and observation of her condition and consider moving her into a nursing home.

WHAT SHOULD MAY DO?

The gerontologist at the hospital gave May a thorough medical examination. He discovered that she was suffering from pernicious anemia (insufficient vitamin B_{12}), hyperthyroidism, and multiple vitamin deficiencies. He immediately organized treatment to restore her nutritional balance and recommended a special diet.

May needs to become better informed about her nutrition requirements, eat well-balanced meals every day, and monitor her health more carefully by visiting the doctor regularly. She should stay in contact with her family and get out of the house as often as possible. Her family should make sure that she is eating properly.

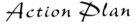

Action Plan

HEALTH
Check weight every week and visit the doctor regularly to monitor any potential problems.

EATING HABITS
Try to eat at least three meals a day and keep plenty of fruit and other healthy snacks on hand for times when eating a full meal is difficult. Cut down on alcohol; eat more fresh fruits and vegetables.

DIET
Have someone help with food shopping and cook and freeze some meals that can be reheated in a microwave when needed.

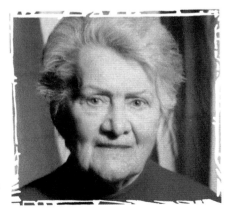

DIET
An inadequate diet can cause nutritional deficiencies that may impair brain function.

HEALTH
Major deterioration can result from not taking personal responsibility for health.

EATING HABITS
Not eating regular, healthful meals can lead to illness that can seriously compromise your lifestyle and independence.

HOW THINGS TURNED OUT FOR MAY

May received treatment at the hospital, which included injections of vitamin B_{12} and supplements of thiamine, and made a rapid recovery. She has been able to resume her reading and is once more enjoying life. Her son's wife invites her regularly for evening meals and takes her shopping, so she always has fresh food at home. May has learned to cook some simple nutritious dishes and is making an effort to improve her eating habits and drink less wine.

senile dementia are in fact suffering from treatable diseases, such as anemia, hypothyroidism, vitamin deficiencies, and urinary tract infections. Mental confusion can appear as a side effect of medically prescribed drugs, especially sleeping pills, sedatives, and antidepressants. Alcohol abuse also depresses the central nervous system.

A good diet is vital for the maintenance and well-being of the nervous system. Deficiencies of the B vitamins, particularly B_1 (thiamine), B_{12}, and folic acid, can affect brain function, causing confusion, irritability, depression, memory loss, and other problems. The antioxidant vitamins, especially E, also play an important role and may delay or prevent senility.

Some people believe that if a deficiency of a nutrient can cause mental problems, extra amounts will enhance brain function. While it is true that a person with a mild deficiency will benefit from increased amounts, there is no evidence that megadoses will be useful; they can even be harmful (see page 87). Supplements should always be taken with the advice of a nutritionist or doctor.

There is at present no known cure for Alzheimer's disease, in which memory, thought processes, and behavior become increasingly impaired. But it does appear that brains that receive a healthy flow of oxygen through good diet and exercise and are stimulated by mental activity are better able to resist succumbing to the disease.

The vitamin-like compound L-acetylcarnitine has shown some promise in delaying the progression of Alzheimer's disease in the early stages and also in treating elderly patients who have memory problems or depression. The hormone dehydroepiandrosterone (DHEA) has been used with some success in treating several age-related conditions, including impaired memory and cognitive functions.

Chess for memory
Chess has been called the king of mind sports. Originating in India, it has been played for centuries and has been enjoyed by well-known people as diverse as Queen Elizabeth I, Tsar Ivan the Terrible, Napoleon, and Benjamin Franklin. The tactical thinking required and the need to remember an opponent's moves apparently aid memory and mind power in those who play the game regularly.

VISUAL MEMORY TEST

A good way to exercise your mind and your powers of concentration is to study an image in great detail and then try to recall as much as possible of what you have seen. Look at this painting for a couple of minutes, then close your eyes and try to remember its details. To test yourself, try answering the questions on page 126. If you practice with different images, you will find your concentration improving.

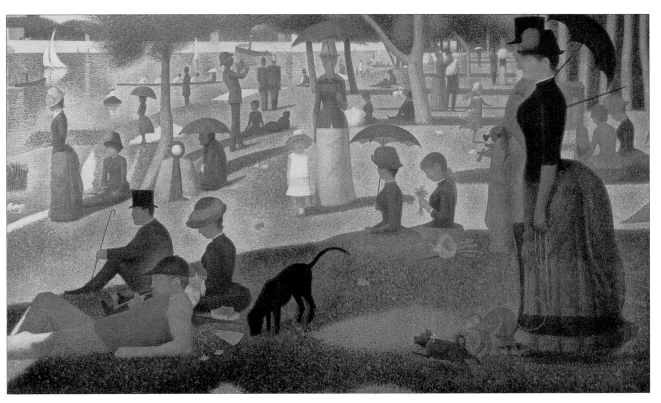

MEMORY TEST

Answer the questions below about the picture on page 125 without looking at it. Don't worry if you can't answer all of them; your concentration will improve with practice.

▶ *Is the picture from the modern day or from another era?*

▶ *What sort of weather is depicted in the picture?*

▶ *Is the season depicted summer or winter?*

▶ *How many dogs are there in the foreground?*

▶ *What is the man in the left foreground doing?*

▶ *Are there more men or more women in the picture?*

▶ *What color dress is the girl in the center of the picture wearing?*

▶ *What is the woman in the right foreground carrying?*

▶ *What animal is being led by the woman in the foreground?*

▶ *How many different types of boats are on the lake?*

HOW TO IMPROVE MEMORY

If you find yourself becoming increasingly forgetful, there are ways in which you can improve your memory. The most immediate, practical thing to do is keep lists, especially when you have a number of tasks that need completing. This will help sort out what you need to do and reduce any concern that you might forget something, because you can check off each item as you have dealt with it.

Your memory can improve with exercise, and there are many aids that you might wish to try. For example, if you are meeting someone for the first time and want to remember his or her name, use a technique called association. Notice something about the person that is striking, such as a facial feature or the way he or she walks or dresses. Connect this with the person's name in your mind. If you make your mental image as colorful and humorous as possible, you are more likely to remember the name.

The Roman orator Cicero used a technique of associating words with images. He developed a system for keeping a mental note of his main talking points by visualizing a familiar building and then putting each theme in a separate place, or *topoi*; this is the derivation of the word *topic*.

Rhyme is another helpful memory device, especially when combined with images. Mnemonic rhymes, such as one for bun or two for shoe, are commonly used.

Repetition is a useful memory tool. The more often you repeat something, the more easily you will remember it. Brain function tests such as PET scans and encephalograms have shown that whenever a mental task is attempted for the first time, there is an increase in the electrical activity and blood flow to the brain. Each time the task is repeated, these changes become less and less marked, indicating that with repetition of a task, the mind needs to exert less and less effort to remember what to do.

MEMORY PROMPTS

There are numerous ways to remember things more easily. Simple lists may work for some, but most people find that using images and color works better. Writing things down in the form of a chart or a flow diagram, with the item you want to remember in the center of the page, will make it easier for the brain to review the information and transfer it to long-term memory. Try relating things you have to remember to unrelated emotions or images to make them stand out in your mind. The chart below contains suggestions for techniques to help you remember anything, from one new name to a long shopping list.

USE YOUR SENSES	USE YOUR HUMOR	USE YOUR IMAGINATION
Synesthesia This is the blending of the senses. If you add sound, touch, smell, or taste to whatever words you are trying to remember, you are far more likely to recall them.	**Exaggeration** Enlarge the size, shape, and sound of any mental images you are trying to remember. This will make the mental image seem unusual and more likely to stick in your mind.	**Color** Make your mental images and written lists colorful and even add pictures of the items on your list. Visual devices usually make things easier to remember than plain text.
Sexuality Most people are interested in sexuality, so using metaphors of romance and passion may help you remember items on a list. You do not have to let anyone know what your memory aid is.	**Wit** The more ridiculous or surreal an image is, the more likely you are to recall it. Remember items by relating them to a comedy television show you saw the previous evening, for example.	**Symbolism** If you have to remember something mundane, try to add images that have more meaning for you. For example, your bank PIN number could be the date you met your spouse.

EMOTIONS AND AGING

Coping well with emotional problems, such as worry and stress, and making your life stimulating and interesting are essential to keeping your mind active, lucid, and healthy.

There is increasing evidence of the importance of a healthy emotional life to both our daily physical well-being and our longevity. But what constitutes good emotional health? Research indicates active engagement in all aspects of life may hold the key.

A long-term investigation by researchers at the Harvard University Medical School in Massachusetts suggested that people who are actively involved in their communities lead longer, happier lives. The project, known as the Grant Study of Adult Development, was launched in 1937. It involved a group of nearly 500 young males from inner-city Boston whose lives, careers, and health records were examined at regular intervals over the course of 40 years.

The head of the research team, Dr. George Vaillant, noticed that the young people in Boston who showed the most successful adjustment to life were those who were sociable, outgoing, and neighborly. When the boys were tested by independent assessors in middle age, it was found that their later development had nothing to do with early differences in intelligence, income, or social class. What mattered most was their level of involvement in their schoolwork, sports, household chores, part-time jobs, and extracurricular activities. Those with the highest activity levels turned out to be the happiest and healthiest adults, the best fathers, and the most successful husbands. As adults they were twice as likely to have built up warm relationships with a wide circle of friends and five times as likely to be in well-paid jobs. And at the end of the study, it was found that their mortality rates were six times lower than those of their less committed classmates.

A firm sense of purpose and commitment also seems to be important in preserving life, as sociologists David Phillips and E.W. King discovered when they carried out a study of New York Jews. The results, published in the *Lancet* in 1988, revealed that Jewish mortality rates showed a marked fall before the Passover but a sharp rise immediately afterward. After testing a number of alternative explanations, the researchers concluded that the excitement of the coming festival helped to prolong life until after the Jewish holiday.

To further test this theory, Dr. Phillips teamed up with another colleague, Daniel G. Smith, to investigate the mortality rates of Chinese people during the week immediately prior to the Harvest Moon Festival. This survey, published in 1990 in the *Journal of the American Medical Association*, examined natural death rates among

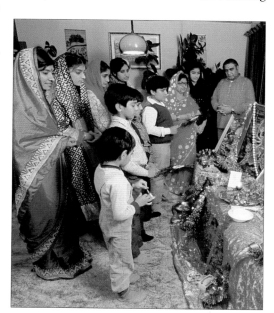

DIWHALI
During the Hindu festival of lights, Diwhali, people gather to celebrate Lakshmi—the goddess of good fortune. Traditions such as these are important, research has shown, because looking forward to a family event or celebration can have a dramatic effect on emotional health, enabling people to resist illness and even postpone death.

Worry not

Abraham Maslow, one of the American founders of humanist psychology, noted that successful, well-adjusted people have the ability to be "lost in the present." They are so absorbed in what they are doing that they forget the cares of the past and have no time to worry about potential future problems. Worry is reduced to manageable proportions once we adopt the practice of living one day at a time.

Chinese families in California from 1960 to 1984. Again it was found that in the week before the Harvest Moon Festival, the Chinese death rate showed a temporary fall of just over 35 percent, only to rise again by the same proportion immediately after the excitement was over. The principles inherent in these findings can be applied to daily life; having a sense of purpose is crucial to well-being, whether it comes from being relied on to stage-manage an amateur theater production or to chair a fund-raising event.

COPING WITH DEPRESSION

Approximately one in every 10 elderly people suffers from depression, which can vary in severity from a mild touch of the blues to deep and dark despair. Depression may be a reaction to physical illness, loneliness, boredom, or a loss of self-esteem. Under the

LIGHT THERAPY

Light allows the pineal gland in the brain to produce natural feel-good chemicals called endorphins. Insufficient daylight during the winter causes depression, or seasonal affective disorder (SAD), in some people. Daily treatments using fluorescent lights that reproduce the whole spectrum of daylight can greatly improve mood.

thrall of depression, life seems pointless and even the simplest task can become an impossible burden. Often low moods are accompanied by physical symptoms, such as chronic fatigue, insomnia, headaches, and loss of sexual drive. As a result, 50 percent of depression cases are missed by doctors. Some are even confused with senile dementia, especially when elderly patients are particularly inactive and withdrawn.

Many depressives take comfort in food. Others seek refuge in smoking, drugs, or heavy drinking, which may provide temporary relief. More effective help can be obtained from self-help organizations, counselors, and psychologists. If the depression is particularly severe, medical help may be needed. But there is plenty that depressed people can do to help themselves.

Depression feeds on itself. Victims sink into a state of apathy and despair, losing all inclination to do anything except sit and mope. The best way to break out of this state is to embark on some course of action. Diversions could include taking a walk, watching comedy films, dancing, listening to music, participating in a sport, or doing a good turn for someone. Even if you don't feel like doing anything, you will feel better once you've taken the first step.

The chemicals in modern antidepressant drugs produce feelings of euphoria because they increase levels of a group of mood-raising substances known as biogenic amines. The best known of these substances is noradrenaline, a naturally occurring hormone produced within the body in response to arousal, excitement, and vigorous exercise. We can get the same effect by following an exhilarating lifestyle, keeping fit, accepting challenges, and embarking on new adventures that give us a break from our routine. Taking a regular walk around your neigh-

QUINDO

Quindo was devised by Khalegl Quinn over 30 years ago to increase vitality, promote relaxation, and relieve depression. Quindo, which aims to give people control over their lives, draws on meditational skills and the defensive martial art of Chi Kung, as well as psychological theory. The exercises are designed to ensure a healthy, protective flow of *chi,* or life energy, through the body. The exercise shown below is called the fountain.

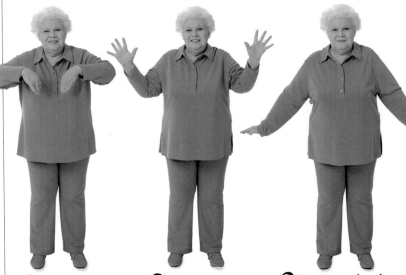

1 *Stand with back straight, elbows raised, feet shoulder width apart, and the backs of your hands facing each other.*

2 *Raise your wrists to chin level and spread your fingers. Move your hands from side to side at the elbow three times.*

3 *Press your hands down below your hips. Pause, slowly repeat the whole sequence nine times, and then relax.*

borhood or participating in a sport may make a big difference to your state of mind. A study carried out at Duke University Medical Center in North Carolina discovered that, irrespective of the severity of depression, those who exercised regularly experienced on average an 82 percent reduction in their feelings of depression.

WORRY AND ANXIETY

Worry is one of the major preoccupations of the civilized world. An investigation of 9,000 Americans conducted by the National Institute of Mental Health revealed that 15 percent of U.S. citizens spend more than half their waking hours worrying. Their brains are in a state of constant agitation, and they hold their bodies tense. As a result, they suffer tension headaches, muscular rheumatism, and back pain. Many of them are permanently on edge, nervous, and irritable. They may take tranquilizers to allay their anxiety and sedatives to help them sleep, and they may seek the help of counselors, but in the final analysis, the worry habit can be broken only by taking steps to develop a more relaxed lifestyle.

Dr. Thomas Borkovec, a professor of psychology at Pennsylvania University, favors scheduling a fixed worry time every day. He has established the Pennsylvania Worry Group and recommends that members set aside a regular time and place for worrying. During the day they are advised to jot down their problems in a notebook. Having done this, they must immediately switch their attention to something less troubling—the completion of an unfinished task, a phone call to a friend, or a walk around the park, for example. They are allowed to dwell on the day's problems only when their scheduled worry period arrives. In this way they gradually learn to reduce the time they spend in worry from five or more hours a day to a maximum of 30 minutes.

COPING WITH STRESS

Stress is an inescapable part of everyday life and has been since prehistoric times. When we are under physical or psychological pressure, our bodies are prepared for action. The physiological changes that take place are exactly the same as those experienced by Neanderthal man. However, the stress experienced by prehistoric people, such as facing a dangerous animal, was generally short-

THE POWER OF MEDITATION

Research into the physical benefits of meditation has shown dramatic results. A study by psychologist Charles Alexander, published in 1989, tested the effects of different types of meditation on nursing home residents whose average age was 81. The participants practiced meditation or mental exercises for 20 minutes twice a day for 12 weeks. Those who meditated had lower blood pressure and better mental health than those who did nothing or played mind games. Interestingly, all those in the meditation group were still alive three years after the study had ended.

MEDITATION FOR LONGEVITY
A 1989 study of the effects of meditation on a group of elderly people showed that those who practiced transcendental meditation on a regular basis lived longer than those who regularly did mind exercises, as well as those who did nothing.

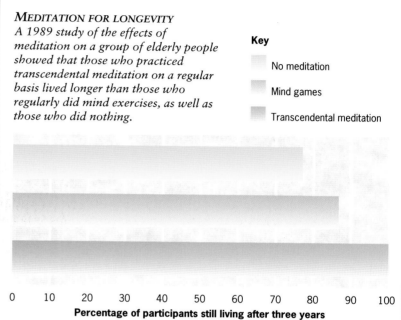

Key

No meditation

Mind games

Transcendental meditation

Percentage of participants still living after three years

lived; the stress faced by people today can be constant. Many people associate dangerous stress levels exclusively with work. However, retirement can also be a time of enormous stress. Adjusting to a completely new way of life without the structure of a regular working day can be very difficult, while changes in income, children leaving home, and health problems are all causes of stress. It is vital to recognize the toll stress takes on health and how relaxation techniques can help to keep us healthy.

A major coronary prevention study funded by the United States government took a sample of 800 men who had already had one heart attack and divided them into two treatment groups. The first group received the standard postcoronary counseling advice: lose weight, stop smoking, reduce animal fat in the diet, and do more exercise. The second group was given advice aimed

Stress relief
Humans are empathetic animals, so when we hear tales of crime, disaster, and civil wars, we often experience the emotions connected with the bad news. One way to lessen this vicarious stress is to take an occasional holiday from global anxiety and despair and focus instead on light-hearted happenings in your own community. Don't dwell on bad news but enjoy more upbeat items. This is not mindless escapism but trying to see life in a broader perspective.

FENG SHUI FOR HARMONIOUS LIVING

Increasingly, people are recognizing that a comfortable atmosphere can improve one's state of mind. Feng shui (pronounced feng shway) is a Chinese art that specifies ways of designing your living space in order to improve the well-being of both your body and your emotions. It is based on the philosophy that your environment should be in harmony with the energy forces, or *chi,* that flow constantly in the natural world. If chi is blocked in any way, it may cause frustration. If it bounces off sharp objects into an area where you sit or sleep, it is known as cutting chi and may cause illness or accidents. Some feng shui techniques for harmonizing the flow of chi within your home are shown below.

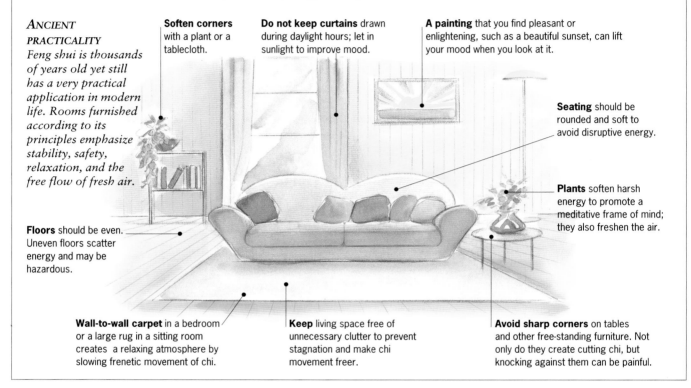

ANCIENT PRACTICALITY
Feng shui is thousands of years old yet still has a very practical application in modern life. Rooms furnished according to its principles emphasize stability, safety, relaxation, and the free flow of fresh air.

Soften corners with a plant or a tablecloth.

Do not keep curtains drawn during daylight hours; let in sunlight to improve mood.

A painting that you find pleasant or enlightening, such as a beautiful sunset, can lift your mood when you look at it.

Seating should be rounded and soft to avoid disruptive energy.

Plants soften harsh energy to promote a meditative frame of mind; they also freshen the air.

Floors should be even. Uneven floors scatter energy and may be hazardous.

Wall-to-wall carpet in a bedroom or a large rug in a sitting room creates a relaxing atmosphere by slowing frenetic movement of chi.

Keep living space free of unnecessary clutter to prevent stagnation and make chi movement freer.

Avoid sharp corners on tables and other free-standing furniture. Not only do they create cutting chi, but knocking against them can be painful.

at helping them to relax. This behavioral conditioning program proved a great success. The men who learned to slacken their pace and laugh at themselves lessened by half their risk of having a second heart attack during the next three years. There are many alternative practices, from meditation to feng shui, that can help you to cope with the pressures in your life.

THE IMPORTANCE OF SLEEP
Sleep is a time of physical and mental renewal. During the night muscles relax, body temperature falls, oxygen consumption drops, metabolism slows, the level of consciousness falls, and the brain becomes calmer; these changes are vital for our bodies to rest adequately and function properly the next day. When we are awake, brain waves are emitted in rapid peaks of 10 or more per second. During sleep they slow down until they become no more than ripples occurring just two or three times a second. During the day body cells are broken down in a process known as catabolism. At night the damage is repaired by the synthesis of new protein molecules, a vital restorative process that is known as anabolism.

Difficulty in sleeping can be a particular problem for older people; surveys show that spells of nocturnal wakefulness become increasingly common as people age. By the age of 45 it is normal to wake up three times a night on average. When this happens, most people immediately fall back to sleep, but others find it difficult. It can help to concentrate on boring things such as spelling words backward or counting sheep. Keeping your eyes open for as long as possible is another tactic; this tires the eyes and evokes the eye-closing reflex that is normally triggered just before sleep.

Making Your Bedroom

A Sleep Haven

To encourage sleep, the conditions within a bedroom should be as similar as possible to those within a mother's womb—soft, soothing, warm, dark, and quiet. The more comforting the environment, the easier it is to enjoy deep, restful sleep.

The reason sleep is necessary is not yet understood; however, it is known that regular sleep is essential for good health. The quantity of sleep an individual needs varies from person to person. Many people suffer from such sleep disturbances as insomnia, which impair their efficiency and can leave them feeling permanently tired and irritable. At the other extreme, many babies and geriatric patients spend most of the day asleep, waking only when they are disturbed, hungry, or in pain.

To promote sleep, the stimuli that keep you awake should be removed. This means no noise, no heavy meals, no late-night worries, no excitement, and no bright lights just before bedtime. Winding down before going to sleep and having a comfortable bed also help.

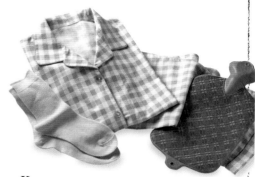

KEEP YOURSELF WARM
The right sleepwear can make a big difference in your ability to sleep. If you have poor circulation, invest in a pair of warm pajamas, bed socks, and a hot-water bottle or electric blanket to keep yourself comfortable.

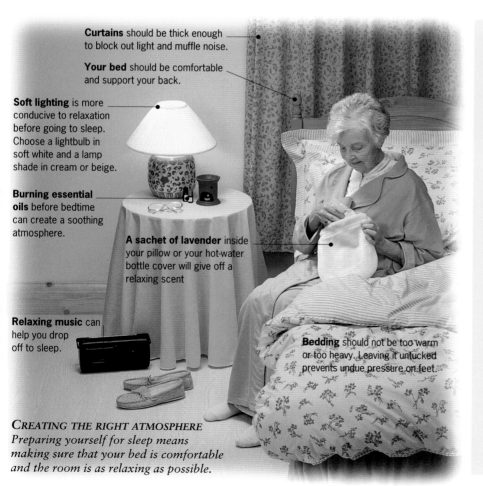

Curtains should be thick enough to block out light and muffle noise.

Your bed should be comfortable and support your back.

Soft lighting is more conducive to relaxation before going to sleep. Choose a lightbulb in soft white and a lamp shade in cream or beige.

Burning essential oils before bedtime can create a soothing atmosphere.

A sachet of lavender inside your pillow or your hot-water bottle cover will give off a relaxing scent

Relaxing music can help you drop off to sleep.

Bedding should not be too warm or too heavy. Leaving it untucked prevents undue pressure on feet.

CREATING THE RIGHT ATMOSPHERE
Preparing yourself for sleep means making sure that your bed is comfortable and the room is as relaxing as possible.

LOBE STROKING

Babies and young children often twiddle their earlobes unconsciously before they fall asleep. This rhythmic action seems to have a relaxing effect because it stimulates a branch of the vagus nerve, which controls the action of the heart and lungs. Researchers working at the Queen Elizabeth Hospital in London, led by Dr. S. R. Saxena, tested the effect of lobe stroking on people ranging in age from infancy to 90 years old. In each case the maneuver produced a slowing of the pulse rate and a marked fall in the strength of the heartbeat and was conducive to sleep. To practice lobe stroking yourself, grasp your earlobe gently between your thumb and forefinger and gently massage it. Do this for two or three minutes or until you drop off.

NATURAL THERAPIES FOR THE MIND

To remain alert, you need enough sleep at night and adequate relaxation during the day. There are many natural ways to calm your state of mind and promote mental agility.

Anxiety, stress, and fatigue can take their toll on the mind. You may be caught in a vicious circle in which depression causes you to feel muddled and forgetful, these states in turn provoke anxiety, and the situation keeps getting worse. Taking time to relax can greatly improve your mental capacity. Such remedies as acupuncture, massage, and meditation not only promote relaxation but can also ensure greater vitality and mental alertness.

Massage
Massage is probably the oldest natural therapy known to humans. We use our hands instinctively to rub, stroke, or knead tense muscles and aching limbs. This action can have a very relaxing effect, as indicated by a study published in the *Nursing Times*. Nurses gently massaged the backs of women who were receiving radiation for breast cancer. Although the patient group was too small to be of statistical significance, the results showed that this simple back massage induced feelings of tranquillity and increased vitality while reducing discomfort, anxiety, and tension. The treatment consisted of gentle effleurage (stroking movements) up the spine, across the shoulders, and down the side of the body to the waist. These types of soothing strokes can be administered by anyone, with little training or experience. Even self-massage—slow, gentle stroking of the forehead, neck, and hands—can have a calming effect. However, better results are obtained from treatment by a practitioner with training in one of the recognized schools of massage, such as Swedish, shiatsu, or Rolfing.

Visualization
Visualization is an effective way to create a positive image that helps you look forward to the future. It is natural for humans to think in images; this is evident in our dreams. Visualization is a way of harnessing this natural ability to create images and expectations in our subconscious, thus setting in motion the possibility of creating the vision.

Scientists believe that our brains are divided into two halves: the left side of the brain is concerned with rational thinking and logic, whereas the right side is creative and intuitive. Most people rely heavily on the left side of the brain and underuse the right. Techniques such as visualization tap into the right side of the brain, which promotes creativity and relaxes the left brain.

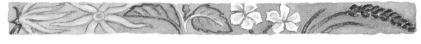

AROMATHERAPY

Essential oils can be used at home in special burners, added to bathwater, incorporated in massage oil, or inhaled. They should never be applied to the skin undiluted, however, as they can be toxic. There are many oils to choose from, but the following are especially beneficial for relaxation and stimulation.

OIL	USE	HOW TO USE IT
Lavender	Antidepressant Relaxing Good for insomnia	Place a couple of drops in bathwater. Place a few drops on your pillow at night. Burn some in an oil burner to scent the room.
Geranium	Mood-lifting Good for insomnia	Add a couple of drops to two tsp of soy or olive oil and massage into your temples.
Ylang-ylang	Relaxant Antidepressant Aphrodisiac	Add one drop to an oil burner. It is a very concentrated and heady oil.
Peppermint	Stimulating Promotes clear thinking Good for treating shock	Add one drop to an oil burner. Do not use at night because it might keep you awake.

Hydrotherapy

Water has always played an important role in natural therapeutics. Beginning in the second century B.C., most major Roman cities contained public baths, or *thermae,* some of which could hold 3,000 bathers at a time. Steam baths have long been popular in Turkey, Russia, and other places, and public bath houses are used widely in Japan as a way to relax and socialize as well as get clean. Stories about centenarians living in the Caucasus Mountains stated they regularly took baths in cold mountain streams.

Bathing can be used both to invigorate and to relax. Cold baths provide a powerful stimulus for the nervous system; they raise the output of stress hormones, deepen the level of respiration, improve blood flow to the brain, and increase metabolism by as much as 80 percent. They also provide a tonic for peripheral circulation, making the smooth muscles lining the walls of the superficial arteries contract, an exercise that has been dubbed "gymnastics for the arteries."

Experiments carried out at the National Medical Institute in London show that human connective tissue cells may be sensitive to temperature change. When maintained in isolated cultures, these cells survive for an average of 57 divisions at normal blood heat of 37°C (98.6°F) but survive for only 19 divisions when the temperature is raised to 40°C (104°F). Cold

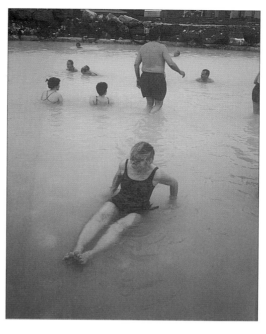

ICELANDIC BATHERS
Icelanders bathe in hot outdoor pools throughout the year to improve their circulation.

showers and baths can provide a valuable metabolic stimulus. If you have a history of heart disease or high blood presssure or are in poor health, however, you should seek the advice of your doctor before taking this therapy; it could be dangerous to take a cold bath immediately after a hot bath or sauna. After taking a cold shower or bath, rub your briskly with a rough towel. This should leave the skin tingling and warm.

Soaking in a warm bath is an effective way to relax. Napoleon apparently soothed his nerves by wallowing in a hot tub. At the onset of war with England, he is reported to have spent six hours in his bath dictating dispatches to his secretaries.

Hydrotherapy is offered in most therapeutic spas and health clubs but can also be enjoyed at home. All it requires is a bath filled with comfortably hot water, containing perhaps a few drops of aromatic oil.

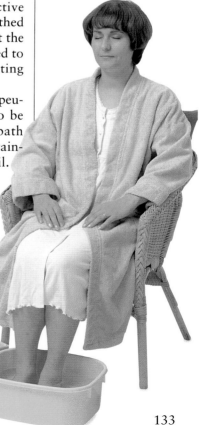

FOOT BATH FOR HEADACHES
Hydrotherapy can be used to relieve a tension headache. Take two plastic tubs and fill one with very warm water and the other with cold water. Sit with your feet in the warm water for 3 minutes, and then plunge your feet into the cold for 30 seconds. Repeat three times, ending with the cold water. Dry your feet thoroughly.

TAOISM

The ancient Chinese philosophy of Taoism embraces many of the ideas that are now advised as essential for improving health and longevity. Taoism is a holistic system that notes the direct effect your physical health can have on your emotional health and vice versa. Taoism sees calmness and being at ease with the world as essential to good health. Taoist scholars instruct their students to "keep a quiet heart, sit as calmly as a tortoise, walk as sprightly as a bird, and sleep as soundly as a dog." They also recommended doing regular exercise and deep breathing, eating plenty of nourishing foods in the winter, and not overeating in summer.

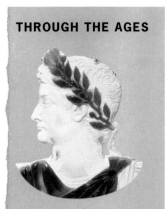

Laurel wreaths
The laurel has long been a symbol of intelligence and achievement. People in ancient Greece put laurel leaves under their pillows to improve their memory and acquire inspiration. The Romans crowned their poets and noblemen with laurel wreaths as a mark of respect. The figure above shows Julius Caesar suitably adorned.

As a precaution, a hot soak should not last longer than 10 minutes; this will eliminate the risk of hyperthermia (a dangerously high body temperature).

Reflexology

Forms of reflexology foot massage have been in existence for more than 5,000 years, although the therapy most commonly used today was developed in the early 20th century. Only the feet are massaged, which means there is no need to undress for treatment, and reflexology can be performed on the frailest individuals without risk of injury, making it especially suitable for older people.

Practitioners of reflexology believe that various parts of the feet correspond to particular organs or parts of the body and thus the whole body benefits from massaging of the feet. Some people find the technique immediately rejuvenating, giving them a renewed spring in their step after each session. Others find it deeply relaxing, so that the massage promotes a deep sleep and greater energy the next day. Another type of reflexology involves massaging the hands.

HERBS FOR MEMORY AND MENTAL STIMULATION

Herbal remedies have been used for thousands of years to treat a multitude of complaints, and many of our conventional medicines are derived from these ancient herbal cures. Some herbs have long been used to improve mental stimulation and relieve the effects of aging. Most of them are relatively safe unless they are taken in excessively large doses. However, it is advisable to consult your doctor before beginning a course of herbal remedies because they can interract with prescription drugs and have a potentially harmful effect on your body.

Ginkgo biloba

Ginkgo biloba was introduced into Europe about 1730, although it was used in China and India for hundreds of years before that. Today ginkgo is among the most widely used of all herbal preparations. It is thought that ginkgo biloba interferes with the platelet activation factor (PAF) in the blood. Among other effects, this prevents blood from clotting, allowing it to flow more freely in the body. Because of this ability to increase blood flow, ginkgo is taken to combat a number of conditions related to aging, including short-term memory loss; it increases mental alertness. Ginkgo is also used to counteract vertigo and tinnitus, common conditions in the elderly, as well as to treat high blood pressure, arteriosclerosis, phlebitis, and peripheral vascular disease.

Most ginkgo products are an extract in pill form. It takes a huge quantity of leaves to make an infusion at home, so it is probably better to choose commercial ginkgo products with a standardized content if you wish to try this herb.

Because ginkgo has an action on blood clotting, it is best not to take it if you have a clotting disorder or are taking hypertension medication. Large amounts of ginkgo have been reported to produce unpleasant side effects, such as irritability, nervousness, nausea, vomiting, and diarrhea.

Ginseng

Like ginkgo, ginseng has a long history in medicinal use and reportedly has a dramatic effect on problems of aging. A controversial herb, it has been the subject of more than a thousand books and scientific papers. Ginseng's supporters claim it is completely safe, acting as a mild aphrodisiac that enhances memory, learning, stamina, and immune functioning. Critics see it as creating a potentially hazardous abuse syndrome, as people may use it to counteract the effects of unhealthy lifestyles. Ginseng can also raise blood pressure and create irregular heartbeats (cardiac arrythmia) and should never be used by anyone with heart problems or hypertension.

It is difficult to prepare homemade ginseng products because the root has to be at least six years old before harvesting and then must be properly dried for at least a month. It is better to purchase a commercial preparation from a reliable manufacturer.

SAGE

Sage has been touted in folk medicine as beneficial for fighting illnesses associated with aging, such as mental confusion, depression, and insomnia. However, pharmacological studies have failed to support these claims, and sage extract and oil are believed to be toxic taken internally on a regular basis. Sage tea, made by steeping 2 tsp dried leaves in 1 cup hot water for 10 minutes, is an effective mouthwash and gargle.

CHAPTER 7

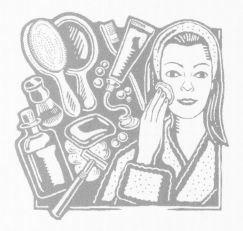

LOOKING GOOD, FEELING GOOD

When you are happy with your appearance, your self-confidence receives a big boost. But what looked good on you in your twenties or thirties will not necessarily flatter you as much in later years. By making adjustments to your wardrobe and hairstyle and paying attention to personal health care, you can continue to be attractive throughout life.

YOUR PERSONAL STYLE

At any time in life, your clothing should enhance your looks by playing up your best points and should reflect your own personal style. As you grow older, what is becoming may change.

In the Western world appearance tends to be very much linked to confidence and self-esteem, whatever a person's age. But images presented by the fashion industry through the media encourage everyone to aspire to particular esthetic standards that are usually of youth, agility, and fitness. Many people therefore associate looking good only with looking younger.

The reality is that every age has its advantages and problems and there is no ideal age, just as there is no ideal image. Some people find that age brings them greater confidence in their looks, and popular culture is beginning to catch on to this idea. After all, a large proportion of the population of Western nations is now over 50. Looking younger is still a goal, but older role models are now challenging this idea.

AGING GRACEFULLY
When men and women make an effort with their appearance, they are not just feeding vanity but are gaining an important psychological boost that makes them feel good about themselves. Looking older is not something you need to be embarrassed about or try to conceal with excessive treatments, lotions, and style changes. Aging gracefully means taking the time to make the most of yourself as you are.

Aging affects the body in various ways. Many people gain weight as their muscle tissue decreases and the amount of exercise they do lessens. Some experience an increase in wrinkles or saggy skin, and most notice a gradual graying or loss of hair. These are all natural aspects of the aging process that may affect grooming and wardrobe choices.

WAYS WITH CLOTHES
There are certain rules that you can apply in choosing your wardrobe to accentuate or camouflage certain aspects of your shape and help project the image that you want.

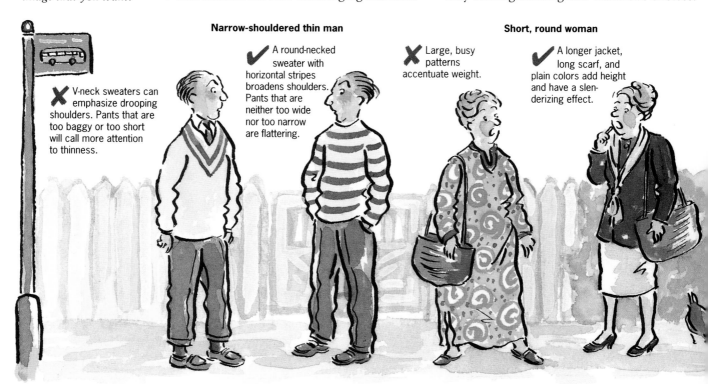

✗ V-neck sweaters can emphasize drooping shoulders. Pants that are too baggy or too short will call more attention to thinness.

Narrow-shouldered thin man

✓ A round-necked sweater with horizontal stripes broadens shoulders. Pants that are neither too wide nor too narrow are flattering.

✗ Large, busy patterns accentuate weight.

Short, round woman

✓ A longer jacket, long scarf, and plain colors add height and have a slenderizing effect.

For example, maintaining a healthy diet and taking the time to moisturize daily can help reduce the impact of aging on the skin. Similarly, getting a new haircut to suit a change, such as acquiring glasses, or changing your cosmetic colors as your skin pales can help you look your best.

YOUR CHANGING WARDROBE

Most people wish to look fashionable but don't want to feel uncomfortable with their image or self-conscious about the way they dress. Wearing the same style of clothing that you wore 20 years ago may make you feel comfortable, but it can also date you and perhaps even elicit criticism from others about your reluctance to grow older.

Instead of reaching for the same old styles and colors, reassess what suits you in light of the physical changes you are experiencing. Gray hair or a paler skin tone, for instance, may allow you to explore a range of colors you previously found didn't suit you. With gray hair and paler skin, there is less contrast in your coloring, and so dramatic, strong colors may be overwhelming. Lighter and neutral or more subdued colors will probably be more flattering. For example, when hair color changes from dark brown to gray and skin tone loses some of its warmth, bright jewel tones that once flattered you may need to be exchanged for more subtle colors, warm pastels, and such neutrals as ivory and gray.

Just as you tried out different styles in your teens, you may need to experiment to revitalize your image as you grow older. Simple changes to your wardrobe do not need to be expensive or drastic. Begin by assessing which of your existing clothes you think really suit you, which have potential, and which need to be sold, thrown away, or given to charity.

Any suit or jacket that is classic, well made, and still fits you can continue to look smart and be easily updated with a fashionable scarf or tie for a more contemporary look. Think about the look you would like to have and make sure that your clothes live up to this image. Above all, remember that your clothes should feel comfortable; if they don't, you will not project self-confidence

It is important that clothes fit properly. Those that are too large or too small are rarely flattering. A jacket should fit well around the shoulders and yet allow free arm movement. Regardless of your shape, a fitted style is generally more flattering because shapeless clothes add visual bulk. On the other hand, a dress or a top and skirt in a knit that drapes subtly over the body, topped by a longer knit jacket, can be more flattering than a close-fitting outfit of woven fabric. Remember, too, any clothing that is too tight will make you miserable.

Women should also adapt their makeup to their skin tone—usually the skin pales with age— and apply it with a lighter touch.

ADAPTING YOUR LOOK AS YOU AGE

Learning to accept the way you are and making the most of your good points can be one of the greatest pleasures—and triumphs—of aging. The following tips can help you enhance your appearance.

▶ *Keep your hair well groomed and have it cut regularly.*

▶ *Look after your clothes and make sure they are stylish and fit properly.*

▶ *Don't wear clothes that are too dated.*

▶ *Wear less makeup and in lighter colors. As your skin becomes thinner and more prone to wrinkles, it is better to adopt a "less is more" attitude.*

▶ *A well-trimmed beard can look very distinguished on a man. Beards and moustaches also protect skin from the sun. A clean-shaven look, however, can be more youthful.*

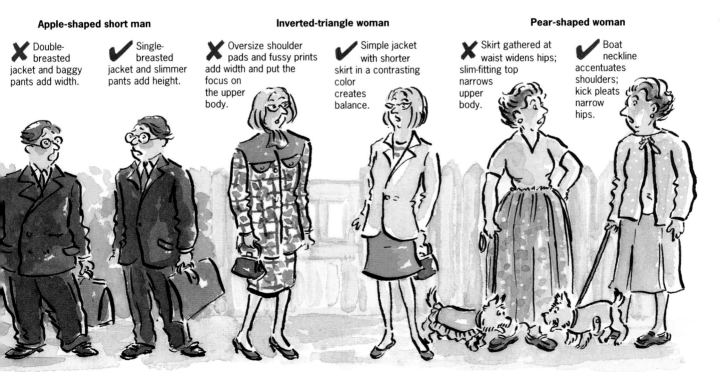

Apple-shaped short man

✗ Double-breasted jacket and baggy pants add width.

✓ Single-breasted jacket and slimmer pants add height.

Inverted-triangle woman

✗ Oversize shoulder pads and fussy prints add width and put the focus on the upper body.

✓ Simple jacket with shorter skirt in a contrasting color creates balance.

Pear-shaped woman

✗ Skirt gathered at waist widens hips; slim-fitting top narrows upper body.

✓ Boat neckline accentuates shoulders; kick pleats narrow hips.

SEASONAL COLORS

Color has the power to affect your mood and how others see you. Some image consultants divide people into color groups. You can consult the categories below to find out which "season" you are, but remember that only fabric swatches held next to your face can reveal which colors are precisely suitable for you.

SPRING

Spring people have pale golden undertones to their skin. Some have ivory skin with freckles; others have clear, creamy skin. The eyes are usually clear and light and have golden flecks in them. Eye colors range from blue and turquoise to hazel and teal. Springs can wear delicate warm colors. These include light orange, peach, all corals, clear and orangy reds, gold, golden yellows, violet, ivory, warm gray, golden brown, clear navy, aqua, clear blue, and pastel or bright yellow greens. Springs should avoid wearing black, silver, and burgundy.

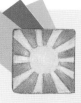
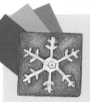

SUMMER

Summer people have pink or blue tones to their skin. They are usually fair, with hair color ranging from pale blonde to ash brown or gray. Their eyes are blue, gray-green, or pale gray. Cool colors are appropriate for summers because they do not have any golden or yellow tones in their coloring. Suitable colors include pastel pinks and blues, burgundy, lemon and other cool yellows, plum, lavender, soft white, pinky beiges, light to medium blues, grays, and silver. Summers should not wear gold, tan, orange, or black.

AUTUMN

Most autumns have warm complexions with golden undertones. They often have auburn, red, or rich brown hair, perhaps with gold or red undertones. They have olive, hazel, teal, topaz, golden brown, or black-brown eyes. Autumns can wear oranges, deep peach colors, rust, terra-cotta, orangey or dark reds, gold, yellow gold, creamy gold, warm beige, camel, brown, blue, turquoise, and olive green. They should avoid wearing any of the cool colors, including blue, forest green, burgundy, purple, and light gray.

WINTER

Winter people have cool coloring like summers, but they are more dramatic. The skin of winter people may be pale or sallow with pink or blue undertones and most have dark hair. The eyes are usually dark: clear hazel, violet blue, deep brown, dark gray, or olive. Winters can wear almost all clean, bright colors, including light and dark pinks, clear and bright reds and yellows, purple, violet, white, taupe, gray, black, navy, and bright greens. They should avoid the warm autumnal colors, such as orange, terracotta, gold, or mustard.

CHOOSING FLATTERING EYEGLASSES

If you have to wear glasses, it is well worth spending time to make sure that they flatter you. If you have a large face, don't wear frames that are too small; likewise, if your face is small, large glasses will overpower your features. Your coloring is also important. If you are fair, avoid dark, heavy frames; if you are dark, light frames may be too strong a contrast.

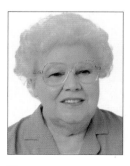

THE RIGHT BALANCE
Match your glasses frames to the size and coloring of your face and hair.

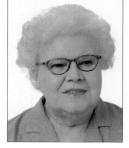

TOO LIGHTWEIGHT
Beware of very small frames if you have a large face; they may make you look bigger.

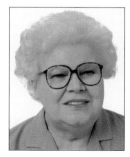

TOO HEAVY
If you are fair, glasses with heavy, dark frames will look overpowering.

Heavy foundation will collect in wrinkles and emphasize rather than disguise them; too much face powder has the same effect. Paler, more muted colors are more flattering than dark or bold colors.

A well-fitted bra to keep the bustline midway between the shoulder and elbow can also make a big difference in your appearance. A poorly fitted bra can cause back and neck pain, and narrow straps can cut into the flesh. It is estimated that as many as 40 percent of women wear ill-fitting bras. Most stores offer a free measuring service, and it is worthwhile taking advantage of it.

GOOD POSTURE

If you adopt better posture, you may be surprised at what a difference it makes in your appearance and feeling of well-being. Not only will your clothes look better because they hang well and sit properly, but you will feel more energetic and ache less at the end of the day. Good posture will also make you look slimmer; if you stand correctly, your muscles will automatically pull in your abdomen, toning themselves as they do. Standing correctly will also lengthen your spine and make you appear taller—some people find they grow as much as 2.5 cm (1 inch). Good posture allows your whole body, including your inner organs, to work efficiently using minimum energy. There is even evidence that correct posture helps to counteract depression.

When you sit down, make sure you don't slump. Sit well back in the chair, so that your back and thighs are supported. If you sit correctly, you will prevent your spine from becoming rounded. Your feet should rest evenly on the floor. Try to get out of the habit of crossing your legs because this inhibits circulation and can cause problems.

Try not to slouch when you are standing. You can use the time-honored technique of walking with a book on your head to develop good posture. Classes in the Alexander technique, a method of adjusting body posture, can also be beneficial. It is important to lift things correctly: keep your back straight and bend your knees (see page 100). If you are carrying bags, balance the weight on both sides of your body. If you carry everything on one side, you put excessive strain on that side, which can throw your hips out of alignment.

SHAPE AND WEIGHT

Many men and women change in shape and put on more weight as they grow older. This is due to a natural reduction in their metabolic rate and often to becoming more sedentary as well (see pages 27–28).

In general, being very overweight is associated with a higher risk of potentially serious health problems, such as high blood pressure, heart disease, diabetes, and cancer. For the 50-plus age group, however, being underweight may be as harmful as obesity. Research in Norway and the United States found that heavier people in the older age groups recovered more quickly from illness and surgery than overly thin people.

The research was based on the body mass index (BMI), which is calculated by multiplying your height in meters by itself and dividing this figure into your weight in kilograms. (To convert from pounds to kilograms, divide by 2.2.) In Canada the recommended BMI for adults up to age 65 is 20 to 25. The U.S. National Institute of Aging suggests a BMI of 22 to 27 for those aged 45 to 55; 23 to 28 for 55- to 65-year-olds; and 24 to 29 for people over age 65.

Some older people find it as difficult to put on weight as others do to lose it. Whether aiming to lose weight or to gain it,

---

CHOOSING THE RIGHT BRA

Wearing the right bra helps to keep a smart figure. A well-fitted bra should lift and separate the breasts and support the bustline midway between the shoulder and the elbow. A badly fitting bra not only will be uncomfortable but also can cause back and neck pain or dig into the flesh and cause bulging. When measuring for your bra size, wear a bra and then use the chart below to find your ideal size.

BRA SIZE				CUP SIZE		
Size in cm	Size in inches	Bra size		Difference in cm	Difference in inches	Cup size
68–72	27–28	32		15	6	B
73–77	29–30	34		17.5	7	C
78–82	31–32	36		20	8	D
83–87	33–34	38		22.5	9	DD
88–92	35–36	40		25	10	E
93–97	37–8	42		27.5	11	F
98–102	39–40	44		30	12	FF
103–107	41–42	46		32.5	13	G

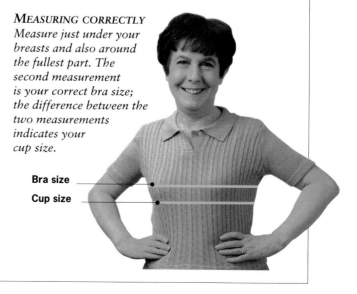

MEASURING CORRECTLY
Measure just under your breasts and also around the fullest part. The second measurement is your correct bra size; the difference between the two measurements indicates your cup size.

Bra size
Cup size

A NEW LEASE ON LIFE

In her youth Lauren Hutton was a successful model and actress but retired when she was 40. However, after her 45th birthday she was asked to model for a New York clothing store. The photographs caused a sensation in the fashion world. It was the first time an older model had been used in a glamorous and appealing way without excessive makeup or picture retouching. Lauren Hutton came to represent a generation of women who felt they had been ignored by popular culture once their "productive" years were over.

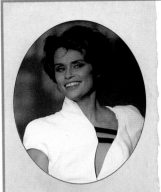

LAUREN HUTTON
In her fifties Hutton became an international model and spokeswoman for breast cancer research.

off instantly. Avoid weighing yourself more than once a week, don't eat separately from your partner or family, and try not to think about food and your diet all the time. This will keep your diet from taking over your life.

Any weight loss or gain should be slow—no more than one to two pounds per week—and sustainable. Rapid increases and decreases in weight have been linked to high rates of illness. Some nutritionists consider it healthier to remain moderately overweight than to swing from fat to thin on a regular basis. Once you have lost weight, you must continue eating healthfully; otherwise, you will put it back on and could find yourself in an unhealthy cycle of yo-yo dieting. As a general rule, if you have kept a consistent weight for two years or more, this is a weight at which your body feels comfortable, and you are likely to remain at this weight for the long term.

You will more readily reach your target weight and will remain in good health if you incorporate regular, moderate exercise into your everyday routine. (See Chapter 5 for more information about how to introduce exercise into your lifestyle.)

Healthy swaps

Swap low-fat foods for high-fat versions whenever possible. For example, have a bagel with a little jam or butter instead of cake or a doughnut; crackers or rice cakes instead of cookies; low-fat yogurt instead of sour cream.

you will still need an adequate intake of vitamins and minerals. Serious health problems can occur when older people do not have a balanced diet (see Chapter 4).

If you do feel the need to lose weight, keep the effort in perspective. Aim for long-term changes and don't expect the weight to drop

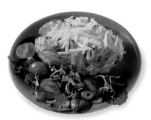

HIGH FAT
A baked potato topped with 60 g of Cheddar cheese has 18 g of fat.

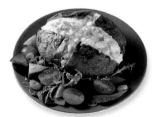

LOW FAT
A baked potato filled with 60 g of cottage cheese and chopped chives contains 2 g of fat.

TIPS FOR IMPROVING BODY SHAPE

Whether you need to lose weight or put it on, certain basic rules apply. Cut down on saturated fats, such as whole-milk dairy products, which can cause heart disease in anyone, no matter what their weight. Reduce your intake of refined sugar, which contains calories but no nutrients.

Do regular, moderate exercise, such as a brisk 20- to 30-minute walk, at least three times a week. Perform sit-ups as part of your morning routine to tone weak abdominal muscles. Always remember to warm up properly before exercising (see Chapter 5 for more information).

TO GAIN WEIGHT	TO LOSE WEIGHT
Aim for a gradual but sustainable increase in weight rather than a rapid rise.	Eat more vegetables and fruits; they are filling and low in calories.
Include more complex carbohydrates in your diet, such as bread, rice, and pasta.	Avoid high-fat snacks. Choose fruit or slices of raw vegetables with low-fat yogurt or salsa dips instead.
If you can't manage large meals, eat smaller portions of nutritious foods at intervals throughout the day.	Choose lean cuts of meat and poultry and remove or drain off surplus fat from food.
Avoid too much saturated fat from fried foods, meat, and whole-milk dairy foods.	Have skim or low-fat milk in hot drinks rather than whole milk or cream and give up sugar in your drinks.
Avoid high-sugar foods, such as candy and cookies, which represent empty calories.	Don't worry about the occasional lapse; be more frugal the next day.
Eat foods high in mono- and polyunsaturated fats, such as nuts, avocados, and oily fish, which are nutritious, as well as high in calories.	Eat dried fruit instead of sweets.
	Drink plenty of fluid with your meals to help you fill up.

SKIN CARE

The skin is often the first part of the body in which you notice signs of aging. Looking after your skin is important not just for your appearance. A healthy skin indicates a healthy body.

Many people feel that changes in their skin are the most visible signs of middle age, but people as young as 20 can find lines developing on the forehead or around the eyes and mouth. The prevalence of wrinkles varies from one individual to another and can be affected by a whole host of external factors, including exposure to sunlight and a person's diet, fitness level, and genetic inheritance. Other skin conditions, such as increased dryness, "liver," or age, spots, and bags around the eyes, can also be age related, although these, too, often depend on a person's lifestyle and may be prevented.

The skin consists of two layers, the epidermis and the dermis. The epidermis is the outer, visible layer that is largely made up of dead skin cells and contains no blood vessels. The deeper layer, or dermis, is composed of a dense fibrous tissue containing elastin and collagen. This layer also contains blood vessels to nourish the skin, as well as muscle fibers, nerve endings, hair follicles, and sweat glands. The layers of skin are attached to the rest of the body by a pad of muscle and fat; this layer provides insulation and protection for the inner organs. Young adults produce new skin cells about every 20 days as their epidermis

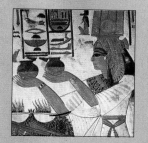
HOW WRINKLES ARE FORMED

The aging process causes the epidermis and fat layers of the skin to become thinner, and dead skin cells are not replaced uniformly when they are shed, causing the outer skin to appear uneven. The inner skin, or dermis, contains the proteins elastin and collagen, which give structure and elasticity to the skin. Elastin fibers normally stretch and spring back, but they become less flexible with age, while collagen fibers develop cross-links, which lock them in place rather than letting them stretch and move with the muscles. The stiff collagen and loose elastin are responsible for the furrows and sags of wrinkled skin.

COLLAGEN FIBERS
Cross-links occur in collagen that block the flow of moisture and reduce elasticity.

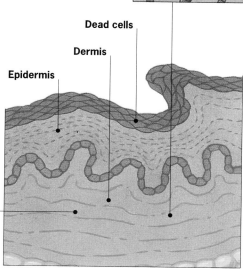

Dead cells

Dermis

Epidermis

ELASTIN FIBERS
Elastin normally springs back into place, maintaining skin tone. As we age, the fibers lose their elasticity, and the skin begins to sag.

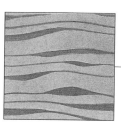

141

Skin cream industry
The fastest-growing segment of the skin care market is for antiaging products. The search for products that will make the skin look younger has led manufacturers back to some of the natural, herbal ingredients, such as chamomile.

sheds dead cells, releases excess moisture, and expels internal pollutants. This cell turnover slows down with advancing age, and the cells themselves often become smaller and less efficient, which is why skin loses its youthful shine and vibrancy in later years. The amount of collagen, the main supporting protein that gives the skin its supple elasticity, also declines, which can lead to sagging. Little can be done to prevent this cumulative effect, but it is possible to minimize external factors to keep skin feeling and looking as healthy as possible. Measures such as not sleeping on the face, always protecting the skin from sunlight, following a healthy, active lifestyle, and practicing a daily skin-care regimen can all help to reduce or at least delay the signs of aging. Performing gentle massage on the face, taking care not to pull or drag the skin, can also tone the muscles, keep them supple, and give you a younger appearance.

WHY WRINKLES OCCUR
Wrinkles are formed by creases in the skin where years of muscle action, such as smiling or frowning, imprint the collagen inside the dermis. Even if you take every precaution to protect your skin, it is almost inevitable that you will develop some wrinkles as you grow older.

Aging occurs in your skin just as it does in any other part of the body, but the skin may appear to age faster because it is so exposed to external pollutants and stresses. Collagen fibers within the dermis keep the skin smooth and taut. Over time these fibers decrease in number and the ones remaining become twisted, hardened, and bound together. It is thought that this happens because of internal and external free radical damage. Once the collagen fibers have hardened, the skin tends to sag and wrinkle, especially in areas where your expressions are habitual—on your forehead or around your mouth, for example.

To guard against free radical damage, eat foods rich in antioxidants (see page 86). Other factors that influence wrinkling are smoking, exposure to air pollution, and consuming excessive amounts of alcohol. These impair your skin's elasticity, as well as its ability to hold water. It is therefore important to eliminate or cut down your exposure to these pollutants. But perhaps the most effective antiwrinkle measure you

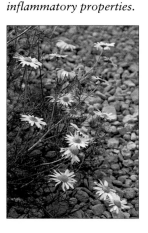

CHAMOMILE
Chamomile flowers contain chemicals called azulenes, which have skin-smoothing and anti-inflammatory properties.

SUN PROTECTION
A prime cause of aging skin is ultraviolet (UV) rays from the sun, especially UVA rays, which also increase the risk of skin cancer. Although it is healthy to obtain some sun—your body needs it to manufacture vitamin D—you should apply a sunscreen with a sun protection factor (SPF) of at least 15 before you go outdoors at any time of year. If you are in the sun for a long time, cover yourself with loose clothing, such as a long-sleeved shirt and pants, and shade your face and neck with a wide-brimmed hat. If you feel a tingling on your skin from the sun, be warned that harm is being done and move into the shade.

can take is to stay out of the sun. It is now proven that sunshine causes 90 percent of all visible skin aging. The sun gives off two types of rays, both of which cause damage. UVA rays go deep beneath the skin, weakening the collagen fibers and causing wrinkles. UVB rays cause burning on the skin's surface and over the years will make the skin look leathery. They also make you more susceptible to skin cancer. Although to some extent sun damage is irreversible, it is never too late to begin taking measures to protect your skin. It is very resilient and will begin to heal itself the moment care is taken. You should protect yourself all year round from the sun. UVA rays are just as penetrative in the winter as they are in the summer.

It is also very important to keep your skin moisturized because wrinkles form more easily when the skin becomes dry. Older people lose liquid faster than those who are

CAUTION
A suntan is your skin's way of protecting itself from damaging ultraviolet rays. About 80 percent of sun damage is thought to occur incidentally, just when walking around outdoors, for instance, so remember to protect yourself with a sunscreen and clothing whenever you are outside.

GIVE YOURSELF A "FACE-LIFT" WITH GENTLE MASSAGE

A regular gentle facial massage is believed to be very effective in helping to keep the skin supple, well toned, and young looking. Start by cleansing the face and then apply a good-quality moisturizer—ideally, one containing vitamin E to counteract free radical damage—and massage the different parts of the face following the sequence shown here. Make sure you are gentle and do not pull your skin too much.

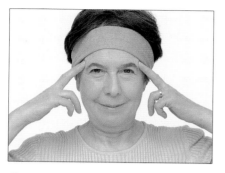

COMBATING CROW'S-FEET
Gently run your fingertips along the outside corners of the eyes; use slightly firmer pressure under the eyebrow but do not pull the skin.

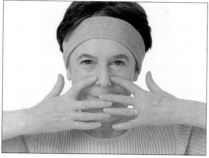

CHEEK TONER
Lace your fingers and press down on your nose and mouth. Gently pull your hands back to your ears over your facial skin. Repeat five times.

CARING FOR YOUR SKIN
Don't pull your skin too harshly during the massage; you could cause more wrinkles to form.

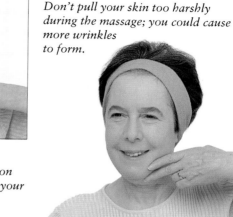

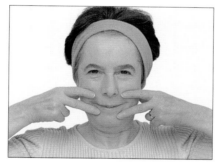

BROW BEATER
Place your fingertips just above your nose and, pressing firmly, run your fingers up to the hairline. Gradually fan your fingers out to the temples.

MOUTH MOVER
Place your fingertips on the corners of your mouth and massage toward your chin, using small circular movements to gently smooth out any wrinkles.

NECK FIRMER
Run your fingers gently along your jaw to your ears, then run your fingers from your jaw down your neck, working from the ears to the center.

younger do (see page 81). Maintaining an adequate water content will help keep the epidermis supple and fresh looking. To do this, it is essential to drink enough fluids—at least eight glasses of water a day. The skin is constantly losing moisture to the air—up to 2 liters (2 quarts) per day. If too much is lost, it can lead to cracking, flaking, and sometimes even chapping. Certain cosmetics, airborne pollutants, and the air temperature and humidity can affect water loss. Regular moisturizing to maintain water balance and consistent care of your skin also help keep the cells regenerating fully so that the skin can function properly.

SKIN CARE PRODUCTS

There is a vast variety of skin care products on the market, and many claim to reduce the signs of aging and provide protection from the ravages of time. By definition, however, cosmetic products are able to treat only the skin's epidermis; any product that penetrates the dermis would be considered a drug and would be subject to strict licensing laws. Despite this, many manufacturers continue to claim that their products have effective, penetrating effects on the skin. The items are often described with confusing, technical jargon that is, in many cases,

continued on page 146

The Dermatologist

The skin is a complex organ that is our primary barrier against infection. It is naturally resilient, but its resiliency decreases with age. Also, skin may become more vulnerable to allergic reactions, infection, and irritation as you grow older.

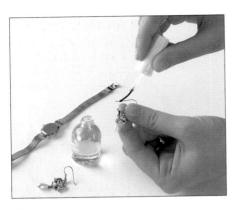

CONTACT DERMATITIS
Developing allergies is not unusual after age 50. Coating watches, rings, and earrings with clear nail polish will help you avoid allergic reactions to metals. You can also back your watch with felt so that the metal does not touch the skin.

Dermatologists are doctors who specialize in the treatment of all types of skin problems. These range from irritating but essentially harmless conditions, such as eczema, to potentially fatal cancerous melanomas. Dermatologists may also detect the presence of other illnesses by observing the condition of the skin in conjunction with other symptoms. For example, an itchy dry skin combined with weight loss and night sweats may be an early indication of Hodgkin's disease and should be referred to a specialist.

What training does a dermatologist have?

A dermatologist is a medical doctor with a good knowledge of internal medicine. He or she has also completed extensive postgraduate training in the treatment of skin disorders.

When should you see a dermatologist?

Patients are usually referred to a dermatologist by their family doctor. If you have a skin condition that concerns you, see your primary care physician first. Dermatologists usually treat long-term skin conditions that cannot be cleared up by a single visit, such as acne or a mysterious itching or rash. They also treat skin cancer and precancerous conditions. Skin disorders should be treated with the same seriousness as other diseases; if you have a rash or other skin problem that has lasted longer than a week, you should seek professional medical advice.

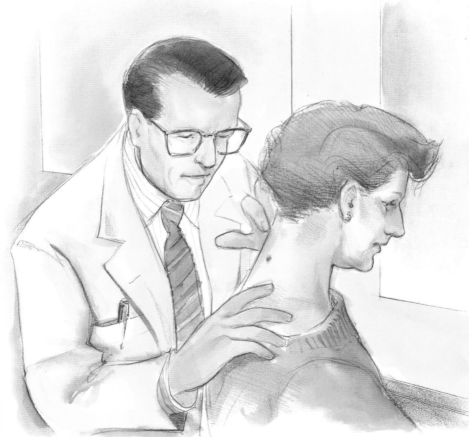

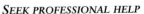

SEEK PROFESSIONAL HELP
Always seek the advice of a dermatologist if you have an unexplained skin condition, such as a mole that has changed its shape, to rule out anything serious. Self-treatment may make a skin condition worse if you do not know the underlying cause.

What will a dermatologist do?

A dermatologist will establish the precise nature of your complaint by thoroughly examining your skin and also asking you questions about the history of the problem. For example, you may be asked when the condition began and whether you are using any medications. Certain drugs, such as diuretics, can make the skin dry, and antihistamines can worsen dermatitis. Some medications can also cause an allergic rash as a side effect. The dermatologist may also ask what you have been eating recently or whether you have changed your soap, because it is common for skin reactions to certain products to develop later in life.

The sudden appearance of a swelling, rash, or hives may be caused by an allergy known as contact dermatitis. Some common culprits are nickel in jewelry, laundry detergents, and synthetic fabrics, any of which may cause severe itching accompanied by patches of redness on the skin. This can be controlled by using bath oils and unperfumed moisturizers and avoiding wearing clothing made from rough materials.

Once a dermatologist identifies your condition and its causes (in the case of allergies, this may take several visits), he or she will prescribe a treatment. This might consist of a topical application or, in the case of an allergy, a list of foods or other potential triggers to avoid.

In addition to dealing with immediate problems, a dermatologist will usually examine the skin all over the body to look for cancerous lesions and precancerous conditions.

What kind of skin problems are older people prone to?

The structure of the skin changes over time, and any of these changes may cause problems. Changes include a buildup of dead cells in the epidermis, increased dryness, and a decrease in pigmentation. The skin may acquire a pallor and a coarser, drier appearance. Also, because of changes in the structure of the epidermis, older skin may become more sensitive to environmental factors and more prone to irritation.

Older skin does not hold water as well as younger skin and has to be moisturized regularly to prevent dryness and flakiness. Flaky skin is more prone to infection, especially if scratched. (Skin infections can be cleared up by applying a prescription cream or lotion.) As we grow older, the glands beneath the epidermis also produce less oil, which may further aggravate any problem.

Some skin problems become increasingly common with age, and others are almost exclusive to older people. One example is rosacea, which often appears after age 40. In this condition the facial skin becomes reddened and may erupt with small blisters. Also, the nose may become red and bulbous. Anything that increases the flow of blood to the surface, such as hot flashes, can worsen the condition.

Aging skin often becomes sensitive to changes in temperature; getting undressed, taking a hot bath, or going outdoors may trigger a severe itchiness called pruritus. This can be

uncomfortable but is not abnormal and should not cause worry. Taking such precautions as avoiding extreme temperatures, dressing warmly, and making sure your home is adequately heated should help relieve or prevent the condition.

Along with a general reduction in hair and skin pigmentation, you may notice isolated dark patches—similar to freckles—appearing on the face and hands or other areas that have been exposed to the sun. These are colloquially known as liver spots. However, they are generally nothing to worry about and should not require any treatment.

WHAT YOU CAN DO AT HOME

As you grow older, your skin needs more care and attention to keep it healthy. Adding oil to a bath instead of using soap, bubble bath, or salts will help prevent your skin from becoming dry and wrinkled. Using glycerin soap or a moisturizing gel in the shower will also help prevent some skin dryness. Apply a moisturizer to your whole body after bathing or showering, more frequently if your skin feels tight. Avoid perfumed products because these can make dermatitis worse.

A little olive oil rubbed into very dry skin, for example, on the elbows, can be soothing. Conditions such as eczema can be effectively treated using homeopathic or herbal remedies; seek expert advice to ensure you get the best treatment.

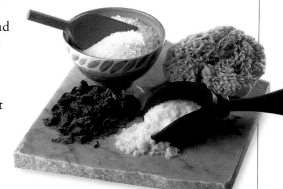

SKIN SOOTHERS
Water can help soothe an itching or irritated skin. Try adding a handful of sea salt to your bathwater and a few strips of dried seaweed (available in most health food stores) or 15 ml (1 tbsp) kelp powder for extra soothing effects. But do not soak for more than 10 minutes.

SKIN CARE FOR MEN

There is much that men can do to protect their skin and help manage aging. Avoid washing the skin too often and use warm rather than hot water and cleansing cream instead of soap, which removes the skin's natural protective oils. Avoid razor bumps when shaving by pulling the razor in the direction of your beard.

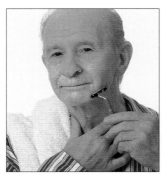

CORRECT SHAVING
Don't stretch your face as you shave because this causes sagging; shave in the direction that the beard grows.

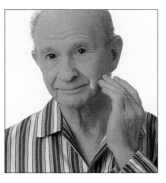

SOFTEN THE SKIN
Apply moisturizer regularly and use emollient (softening) creams on skin made dry or rough by the wind and cold.

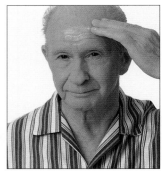

PROTECT THE SKIN
Apply sunscreen to exposed skin, such as the face, ears, back of the hands, and if necessary, the scalp.

entirely meaningless. Skin, in fact, regenerates itself from the inside out, and no external application can actually alter its cellular process. While it is very unlikely that there will be a miracle cure for the natural processes of aging, there are some products that, if used regularly, can help to minimize damaging effects and keep skin as healthy and young looking as possible.

Moisturizers

The term *moisturizer* is a misnomer because such a product does not usually increase the skin's water content but instead helps to seal in and maintain existing moisture levels. Products that help seal in moisture may also stimulate cell reproduction and general skin health. While most moisturizers only maintain the humidity of the epidermis, some claim to be hygroscopic, or water attracting. These products work by literally pulling water from the air to keep the exterior skin layer supple and moist. Many rely on a concentrated solution of Na-PCA, a naturally occurring chemical in the skin that gradually declines with age. It is thought that when its water content is maintained at a consistent level, the epidermis will remain soft and cushioned, thus limiting the depth of furrows and wrinkles that develop.

Vitamin-enriched products

Vitamins, which have long been heralded as essential for good health and vitality, are now often featured in skin care preparations. Vitamin E, when applied to the surface of the skin, helps protect the cells from damage caused by exposure to UV light or chemotherapy. Vitamins A and C, along with the trace elements zinc and selenium, are thought to enhance the skin's natural healing process by stimulating epidermal cells. Skin that continues to replenish itself properly will therefore look better, with a smooth, contoured texture and glowing, fresh exterior.

Even essential fatty acids (EFAs) can be applied to the skin to increase the skin's moisture-holding capacity and encourage a

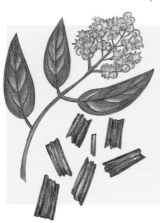

SANDALWOOD AFTERSHAVE MOISTURIZING BALM

In a double boiler melt 10 g (⅓ oz) beeswax with 25 ml (2 tbsp) jojoba oil. Remove from the heat and drizzle 80 ml (⅓ cup) elderflower tea into the oils, blending with a whisk until an emulsion is formed. Cool slightly, then blend in 10 drops essential oil of sandalwood, 8 drops cedarwood oil, 8 drops bergamot oil, and 4 drops tincture of benzoin. Store in a clean jar.

better exchange of nutrients between the cell walls. There is some debate among scientists as to whether external application of vitamins and EFAs can be as effective in aiding skin quality as taking them internally as part of a healthful diet. Even so, many cosmetic companies are including these nutrients in their products with the promise of helping to restore tired-looking skin.

Alpha hydroxy acids (AHAs)

Alpha hydroxy acids, found abundantly now in a variety of skin lotions, are a natural way of exfoliating dead skin cell layers. The main types of AHAs used for this purpose are malic, derived from apples; lactic, derived from milk; glycolic, coming from sugar cane; and pyruvic, derived from papayas. They work by gently dissolving the intercellular glue that makes old skin cells stick to the epidermis. AHAs help to refine the external layer of the skin, making it look brighter, finer, and better at refracting light. Some dermatologists believe that the acids can also enhance the skin's moisture-holding ability, so that the tissue maintains its soft, padded firmness.

USING THESE PRODUCTS

While you cannot reverse the changes in your skin, you can inhibit some of the processes that cause damage. The sooner you start taking care of your skin, the healthier and more vibrant it will be. Ideally, daily moisturizing and a consistently healthy lifestyle from a young age have kept your skin in good condition, so that hardening of the collagen and reduction in skin moisture have been delayed.

MAKEUP

While some makeup can dry skin and clog pores, experts believe that most good-quality products provide useful protection by holding in existing moisture and deflecting UV rays and pollutants. Choose hypoallergenic products, which are less likely to cause irritation, and remove them completely every night. Carefully chosen makeup applied with care can enhance your appearance.

VITAMIN C FACE PACK
Crush one 1,000 mg vitamin C tablet in a small bowl. Stir in 1 tsp orange blossom water (available from pharmacies). If using an effervescent tablet, wait until the fizzing subsides, then add 1 tsp of powdered green clay (available from herbal suppliers) to make a smooth paste. Blend in 1 tsp almond oil and 2 drops orange oil. Smooth over your face, avoiding the eyes and mouth. Leave for 15 minutes and then rinse off. Refrigerate any remainder and use within a week.

SURGICAL TREATMENTS—PROS AND CONS

Surgery is sometimes the only way to repair certain effects of aging. However, such treatments are expensive and painful and may be short-lived. Before deciding to have surgery, make sure you understand what is involved, the cost, the success rate, the time required to recuperate, and any associated risks.

TREATMENT	HOW IT WORKS	PROS AND CONS	LASTS FOR
Dermabrasion	Upper skin layers are scraped off to remove freckles, liver spots, acne scars, blemishes, and superficial wrinkles.	Encourages new skin growth; does not remove deep wrinkles; may take weeks to heal; may be painful.	Several months
Collagen implants	Collagen, a protein extracted from cattle, is injected under the skin to fill depressions, wrinkles, and minor scars.	Has few long-term side effects; may be painful; is not effective on sun-damaged skin	6–12 months
Cosmetic surgery	Various surgical techniques are used to remove, redistribute, or reshape tissue to fill or tighten wrinkles and sagging skin. Materials like silicone, synthetic paste, or body fat are used to fill hollows and creases.	Usually long lasting and highly effective; risk of serious side effects is high; procedures are expensive.	Several years

CASE STUDY

An Insecure Woman

A change in lifestyle, such as children leaving home, can have a dramatic effect on a woman, especially if she has neglected her appearance. A new haircut and some new clothes may seem like frivolous expenditures, but they can have an important effect on mental health and set up a positive beginning to a new phase in life.

Susan, 50, is the mother of two children who have recently left home. Susan's husband, Fred, wants to socialize more and meet some new people now that they have more time together. With the children no longer the focus of her life, Susan has recently become uncomfortable with her appearance. She usually dresses in leggings and baggy sweaters. Her hair has become very gray, and she has not had it cut for a couple of years. She has also gained a lot of weight and has noticed some shadowing on her upper lip. Her lack of confidence in her looks makes her dread evenings out. When she and Fred were first married, she was confident and outgoing, but now feels shy, insecure, and old before her time.

WHAT SHOULD SUSAN DO?

Susan should not feel that she has to look spectacular in order to have a good time, but taking a little more care with her appearance will bring an important psychological boost. She should first look at losing weight and increasing her fitness. Her doctor provided a few guidelines for weight loss, such as eating low-fat foods and plenty of fruits and vegetables. He also suggested that she do some regular exercise. In order to motivate herself with her new routine, Susan could go to the hairdresser for a new haircut and possibly new color, which would provide an immediate lift. Now that she has more time to socialize, she could consider investing in some new clothes.

Action Plan

CLOTHES
Don't wait until excess weight is lost before buying some simple and flattering new clothes. Wear them immediately.

GROOMING
Invest in a flattering haircut and perhaps some other beauty treatment to boost self-esteem.

LIFESTYLE
Resolve to lose weight and regain fitness. Participate in community activities and social events. Focus on helping others to avoid self-consciousness about appearance.

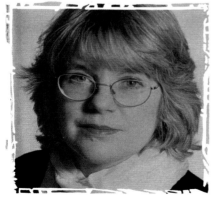

LIFESTYLE
When a role changes, insecurity often translates into dissatisfaction with other areas of life.

CLOTHES
As self-esteem drops and weight begins to increase, many people try to hide themselves in baggy, unflattering clothes.

GROOMING
Neglecting appearance can lead to lack of self-confidence in social situations.

HOW THINGS TURNED OUT FOR SUSAN

Susan began by eating sensibly and taking long walks every day. She had her hair cut in a shorter, more manageable style and colored a flattering reddish brown. She felt relaxed enough at the salon to book herself for a facial. Recently she bought herself a new dress to wear to an upcoming party and another one in a smaller size to wear later. Even before losing any weight, Susan was beginning to feel much more confident about her looks.

TEETH AND HAIR

Keeping yourself well groomed and attractive involves more than just skin care. Looking after your teeth and keeping your hair healthy and clean are vital to your appearance.

Opinions differ over how much the progress of time affects teeth. Years of chewing do wear down tooth surfaces, but as long as the mouth is properly maintained, most dentists today believe that there is no reason why anybody should have to undergo any drastic dental treatment. Many people have accumulated fillings, crowns, or some kind of dentures by middle age, but the likelihood of needing these can be minimized by taking good care of your teeth throughout your lifetime.

Dental care

There is no alternative to careful daily brushing and flossing of the teeth, along with regular visits to a dentist and hygienist. It is essential to brush and floss your teeth at least twice a day, even more often if you have the opportunity. Use a soft toothbrush rather than one with hard bristles, which can damage your gums and tooth enamel. Apply a pea-sized blob of toothpaste to the brush and brush the teeth in a circular motion, concentrating on the gums. Make sure you reach the back of your mouth and behind your teeth and that you brush for at least two minutes. To floss your teeth, take a length of floss at least 30 cm (12 inches) long and wind it around your index fingers. Floss gently in between each tooth, removing trapped food debris and plaque. Then rinse your mouth.

AGING AND YOUR TEETH

The term "long in the tooth" has often been used to describe advancing age. This is because levels of collagen decline, causing gums to recede and more of the tooth to be exposed. The newly exposed part of the tooth is particularly vulnerable to plaque and tartar because it lacks a protective layer

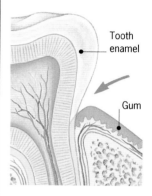

INSIDE A TOOTH
Bacteria can easily invade the area where the gum and tooth meet, shown here by the arrow. The bacteria attack the tooth enamel and cause decay.

CORRECT BRUSHING AND FLOSSING

To prevent tooth and gum disease, brush your teeth at least twice a day. Use a fluoride toothpaste and remember to brush the top and inside of each tooth. Use gentle circular motions and make sure you brush your gums as well as your teeth, paying particular attention to the area where your teeth and gums meet. Gently move the brush backward and forward using small strokes.

Ideally, you should floss your teeth every time you brush. Be sure to include the back teeth and the teeth adjacent to any bridgework because this is where food debris and plaque can accumulate. Instead of dental floss you could use a battery-operated water pick that squirts a thin jet of water between teeth.

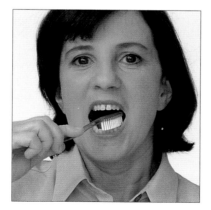

HOW TO BRUSH
Place the brush at a 45-degree angle to your gums and make sure you brush all areas, including the back teeth, all the surfaces, and the gums.

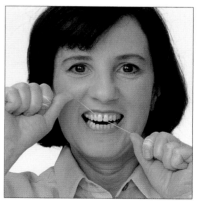

HOW TO FLOSS
Snap off a generous length of floss and curve it around each tooth, gently sliding it along the tooth to the gumline and back again.

Easy-grip toothbrushes

If you find it hard to grip your toothbrush to use it effectively, try one of these inexpensive ways to make life easier for yourself.

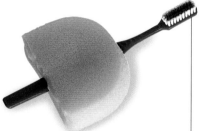

LONG LENGTH
Extending the length of your toothbrush handle by taping lollipop sticks to it can make the tooth-brush easier to hold if your arms are not supple.

SPONGE GRIP
Inserting the toothbrush handle into a piece of foam or a sponge makes it easier to hold if your hands are stiff or you suffer from arthritis and find it hard to grip.

DENTURE CARE

Your gums naturally recede with age, which means that if you wear dentures, they may fit less well over time and have to be altered or replaced. Taking care of your dentures is always important, however. Below are some tips.

▶ *Have dentures and bridges checked by a dentist at least every five years.*

▶ *Clean dentures every day to avoid disease that can affect gums and remaining teeth.*

▶ *Soak them thoroughly according to your dentist's instructions.*

▶ *You should also brush dentures regularly to prevent a buildup of plaque, which may attack your gums.*

▶ *When cleaning your dentures, pay particular attention to the edges and the spaces between the teeth.*

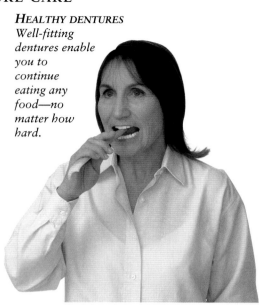

HEALTHY DENTURES
Well-fitting dentures enable you to continue eating any food—no matter how hard.

---

of enamel to cover the soft layer of dentine beneath. If plaque is allowed to build up and eat away at the dentine and connective tissue, the tooth will become loose and may eventually require extraction. Unfortunately, gum disease affects about 95 percent of adults, usually in the form of bleeding gums. Gum disease is the main contributor to tooth sensitivity, damage, and loss. This is why it is particularly important to maintain good regular dental hygiene.

If you do lose a tooth or chip one, it is important to take action quickly. Teeth hold each other in place; if one goes, the others may change position or become loose. Dentists have a number of methods for filling such spaces to protect the remaining teeth. You should have a denture or bridge fitted to fill large gaps, or the adjacent teeth will spread to fill the space, causing more gaps and weakening the connection between the teeth and jaw.

Dentures, implants, and crowns

Dentures can consist of a few false teeth held together by a bridge, or a complete set for both the upper and lower mouth. They should be washed and cared for with nightly soakings and regular hygiene (see box, above). The mouth continues to change shape with age, so most dentures have to be replaced every few years to avoid straining the jaw or even causing possible ulceration.

Dental implants are more akin to real teeth and are usually more expensive than conventional dentures. With the patient under anesthetic, tiny metal cylinders made of lightweight titanium are surgically implanted into the jawbone. A thin metal post is then screwed onto the cylinder and left for six months to allow bone to grow tightly around the implant. When the post is securely set in the mouth, an artificial tooth is mounted onto it.

Crowns, or caps as they are sometimes known, are used to cover a decaying tooth to protect it from further erosion or prevent any mishaping of the mouth. They are made of metal or porcelain and are cemented onto what remains of an existing tooth.

Whiteners and veneers

Years of eating, drinking, and smoking can cause stains and discoloration of the teeth. Tiny cracks in the enamel soak up coffee, black tea, wine, tobacco, and various food dyes, leading to a gradual yellowing of the enamel and general dullness in color of the teeth. It is possible to reverse some of these changes, but most experts do not recommend commercial tooth whiteners because they often contain caustic chemicals that damage the enamel even further. Special bleaches can be used on teeth that have mild stains, but these do not seal cracks in the enamel, so discoloration often returns.

If discoloration is very unsightly, a dentist can cover a tooth with a thin porcelain veneer that is custom-made to fit the tooth. After the front, sides, and underside of the tooth are etched with a mild acid, the veneer is fastened with a strong resin. This protective layer should last for up to 10 years. Veneers can also be used to cover small chips in the teeth, preventing the need for a crown.

SCALP TONIC
Pour 500 ml (2 cups) of cold water into a pan and add 4 tbsp each fresh or 2 tbsp each dried rosemary and chamomile. Bring to a boil, then simmer for 30 minutes. Remove from the heat and leave for at least 1 hour with the lid on, then strain. Stir in 1 tsp borax until dissolved. Pour into a 500-ml (1-pint) opaque bottle to keep out the light and add 5 drops each of bay, cedarwood, lavender, and lemon essential oils; shake well. Store in a dark place. Very gently massage a few drops of the mixture into your scalp every day.

HAIR
Changes in hair are often the most visible signs of aging. Whether it is hair loss or graying, people tend to recognize these changes as an indication of progressing age and a sign that the body is slowing down, even though some people begin to go gray or bald as early as their early twenties and thirties. In fact, like wrinkles, changes in the look, condition, or amount of hair can result from a number of factors. Lifestyle, hormone levels, and genetic inheritance are as likely to determine when such changes occur as the onset of natural aging.

Hair loss
The average person loses about 100 hairs every day as the body creates and sheds new strands as part of its regenerating cycle. Permanent hair loss begins when some hair follicles wear out and are not replaced, so that fresh strands of hair are not generated.

The rate of loss is genetically determined, but the exact cause remains a mystery.

Many experts believe that there is a connection between hormonal changes in the body (particularly in testosterone) and follicle reproduction. Although natural hair loss is more pronounced in men, women also experience a thinning of hair on the crown, which often begins around the time of menopause, when estrogen levels drop. This also explains why a number of younger women experience hair loss when pregnant.

Temporary hair loss can be caused by illness, certain drugs, and nutritional deficiencies, particularly a lack of vitamin A and the minerals iron and zinc. In all these cases hair normally grows back when the problem is

Cures for baldness?
Cleopatra advised Julius Caesar to apply a concoction of horse teeth and burned mice and deer droppings to prevent baldness. The French are said to have advocated potions of alcohol and beef; the Germans, extract of bovine heart; the Hungarians, horseradish and mustard oil. Balding Japanese would strike the scalp 200 times a day with a special brush.

PROTECTING YOUR HAIR

About 30 percent of a hair follicle is water, which is essential to maintain strength and elasticity. The outer surface of the follicle is protected by an oily secretion called sebum. You can help to reduce hair loss by keeping processes such as coloring, bleaching, and permanents to a minimum because these tend to dry the hair and cause damage. Use a mild shampoo and lather only once. Apply a protein conditioner to repair damage and help replace the hair's moisture. Dry your hair using only medium heat; leave it slightly damp. Do not use a sharp nylon brush and remove tangles from long hair by working from the ends toward the roots. Rinse out any salt or chlorine after swimming.

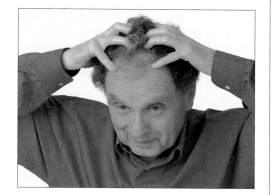

GENTLE SCALP MASSAGE
Massaging the scalp increases blood flow to your hair. Use the pads of your fingers or the flat of your hand to gently move the skin of your scalp over your skull. Do not move your fingers on the skin, as you could pull hair out.

UPSIDEDOWN
Standing on your head is claimed by some to prevent baldness. It may increase blood flow to the scalp, but has not been proven to stimulate hair growth.

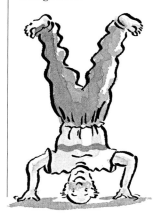

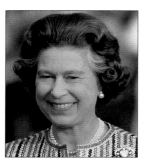

GRAYING GRACEFULLY
You can use your gray hair to advantage. Sweep the lighter hair on the sides of the face up to draw the eye upward, which will give your face a younger look. This style has been used by a number of well-known women, including actress Elizabeth Taylor and Queen Elizabeth II.

rectified, so if you are experiencing hair loss, it is well worth consulting your doctor to investigate the cause. Little can be done, however, for genetic hair loss. If this is causing you distress, you may wish to consider some kind of hairpiece. These can be worn to cover the entire scalp or put over a balding patch and blended in with the remaining hair. It is best to get professional advice when buying a wig or toupee to ensure that it blends in properly with your existing hair and suits your face and style.

Some hairpieces are attached permanently to the head. They are tied or glued to existing strands, or in some cases strands are implanted in the scalp, although this process does carry a risk of infection. Wigs and clip-on extensions are usually the best option because they can be brushed and washed thoroughly and removed to allow the scalp to breathe. Even so, prolonged wearing of a wig can lead to further hair loss because the heat and lack of airflow to the scalp seem to cause scalp disorders.

Hair color

Just as the number of functioning hair follicles decreases with age, melanocytes—cells that produce pigmentation—also diminish and deteriorate. Less pigment is secreted into the base of the hair follicle until the emerging hair appears as a pure white shaft. Although we refer to this process as graying, the strands produced are actually completely white; it is the surrounding hair that makes them look darker in color.

Many people choose to color their hair to cover the gray, either with permanent dyes that remain until the hair grows out or with temporary rinses that wash out over the course of a few weeks. If you just want to liven your hair color and provide gentle conditioning, there are a number of herbal rinses that you can apply. These can darken the gray or give your hair a glowing, silvery shine. To make a rinse, add the desired herb to a bowl of boiling water and steep until it is cool. After washing your hair as usual, lean over a bowl, perhaps placed in the bathtub or a sink, and use a pitcher to rinse your hair with the herbal mixture, catching the liquid in the bowl. Keep repeating this process as long as you can—until your arms ache or you have lost most of the mixture through splashing. The results will not be instant or restore your natural color but will build up over a period of weeks or months.

If you have gray hair, try a rinse made from betony, marjoram, rosemary, or sage. For dark hair, you can use comfrey, marjoram, raspberry leaf, rosemary, sage, or thyme. For red hair, rinse with marigold flowers, ginger, or saffron. You can also use henna, but it is not advisable if you have any grey in your hair. For blonde hair, use a chamomile rinse.

REMOVING UNWANTED HAIR

Unwanted hair tends to become a problem with advancing age. On women it is facial hair that grows on the upper lip. On men hair grows in the nose and ears. There are ways to remove or disguise unwanted hair, but follicles will regenerate new strands. Electrolysis permanently removes hair but is expensive and takes several attempts.

TREATMENT	HOW IT WORKS	PROS AND CONS	LASTS FOR
Depilatory cream	Cream is applied to the skin and dissolves hair just below the skin surface.	Quick, easy, and painless; may cause a rash on some people; test before applying to face.	2 weeks
Wax	An area of skin is coated with wax. Once dry, the wax is peeled away, pulling the hairs out by the roots.	May inhibit regrowth; painful; making sure skin is warm and moist can help reduce pain.	2 weeks, longer in some cases
Tweezers/ scissors	Individual hairs are snipped off or pulled out at the roots.	Painful; use astringent to make hair easier to grip.	As above
Electrolysis	A sterile electric needle is inserted into the hair follicle and a charge is applied. Over time the follicle stops regenerating and the hair stops growing.	Long-lasting; highly effective; slow process; may require a long course of treatment, which can be expensive.	Years; may eventually be permanent

FOOT CARE

*We walk some 120,000 km (75,000 miles) during a lifetime,
so it is not surprising that feet tend to show wear and tear.
Good foot care is vital to feeling well and looking good.*

The skin covering the feet thins over time because of decreasing levels of collagen (see page 142), and this may result in aching or painful feet. Painful feet can have a profound effect on your well-being, causing posture problems and back, knee, hip, or neck pain. They can even cause tension that leads to headaches.

From your thirties onward, the feet will spread—a natural process called splaying. Ligaments in the foot begin to collapse, the arches fall, and the feet become flatter. These changes cause problems because they happen so gradually. People don't notice their feet changing shape and continue to wear the same size shoes, which become tighter and cause pain and such problems as corns or bunions in later life.

A change in body weight also puts strain on the feet. The fatty pads on the balls of the feet become thinner over time. Soft-soled shoes and cushioned insoles are excellent ways of compensating for this. Shoes need to fit comfortably, with about 1.5 cm (½ inch) between the big toe and shoe tip. Moderately low heels with a broad base across the instep also provide feet with suitable support and enable the blood to circulate adequately. Women who often wear shoes that are backless may suffer aching feet because the only way they can keep the shoe on is to grip it with the toes. This type of shoe should be worn only in situations where little walking is required. For appearance's sake, many people buy shoes that are too tight, but it is not attractive to look uncomfortable and in pain. Shoes that are too tight not only are uncomfortable but also may lead to more serious problems. On the other hand, they should not be too loose because they won't support the foot.

People who do a lot of walking and suffer hot, aching feet should consult a podiatrist, who can advise on suitable shoes and recommend treatment for a specific foot disorder.

Problems with the feet

Corns, a buildup of dead skin usually caused by shoes that do not fit properly and that exert extra pressure on the skin, often appear on the joint of the toe or under the surface of the foot. They can be very painful

continued on page 156

LIMITING INFECTION

When dealing with fungal infections like athlete's foot, it is important to prevent spreading of the disorder. Always use a separate sponge or washcloth and towel for the affected parts, change your socks or stockings daily, and spray the insides of your shoes with disinfectant. If you touch the affected area, wash your hands before touching any other part of your body.

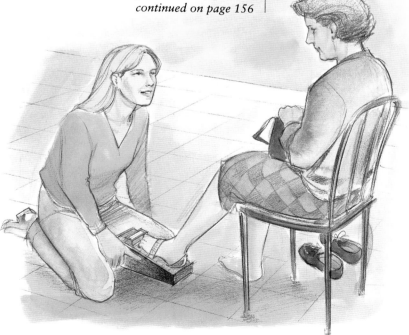

*IDEAL FOOTWEAR
Making sure that your shoes are fitted properly and that they provide adequate support will help your feet stay healthy and pain-free for your lifetime.*

153

The Podiatrist

The feet are a vulnerable and often neglected part of the body. Poor foot care and a reluctance to have a foot disorder treated promptly can lead to debilitating problems. A timely visit to a podiatrist can prevent complications and unnecessary pain.

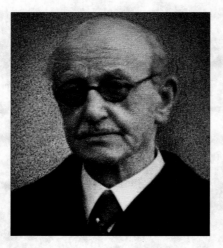

CLUES IN YOUR SHOES
A podiatrist can tell a lot about your feet and posture by looking at the way in which your shoes wear down.

Podiatrists are medical professionals who specialize in the prevention, diagnosis, and treatment of foot and lower limb disorders that result from disease or injury. The name *podiatrist*, which is used in all English-speaking countries, has now largely replaced *chiropodist*, which was in common use for many years.

What do podiatrists treat?
Podiatrists treat a wide range of foot disorders. These include infections, ingrown toenails, corns, calluses, nail diseases, heel spurs, and foot ulcers. They also treat deformities, such as flat or weak feet, foot imbalance, and incorrect walking patterns, often by designing or fitting corrective inserts (orthotics), mechanical devices, and casts. These specialists are trained as well to deal with ankle and foot injuries, which are common among athletes and dancers. By age 70, four out of five people have developed foot problems, so podiatric care is especially important for older people.

Podiatrists also play a vital role in regular preventive foot care for people who have diabetes and circulatory problems. Anyone with these conditions is at a high risk for developing foot infection and complications, such as foot ulcers and gangrene (tissue death), if a foot disorder is not recognized and treated at the earliest opportunity.

Origins

Before chiropody was organized as a medical discipline, problems concerning the feet were usually dealt with by general practitioners, surgeons, or nonmedical doctors. The first society of chiropodists in Europe was founded by Ernest Runting and Arnold Whittaker Oxford in 1912. They agreed that a professional society should be set up to protect the public from charlatans. The Pedic Clinic on Silver Street, London, opened in November 1913. The clinic treated the poor and trained foot orderlies for duties in the First World War. The Pedic Clinic became the London Foot Hospital, and the first school of chiropody opened there in November, 1919. During World War I, other centers were set up

ERNEST RUNTING (1861–1954)
One of the pioneers of education and training in chiropody, Runting helped to establish the discipline.

nationwide. This network of societies was combined into the Society of Chiropody in 1945. Since that time, similar societies have been established worldwide.

With whom do podiatrists consult?
Because foot problems can affect walking, they often cause secondary disorders in the back, hip, knee, and ankle. Podiatrists are trained to recognize these complications and refer a patient to another medical professional, such as an orthopedic surgeon—a doctor who specializes in the treatment of bone and joint disorders. Because the foot often reflects what is going on in the rest of the body, it may be the first to reveal signs of heart disease, kidney disease, arthritis, or diabetes; thus a podiatrist is in a position to spot these symptoms and refer a patient to an appropriate specialist.

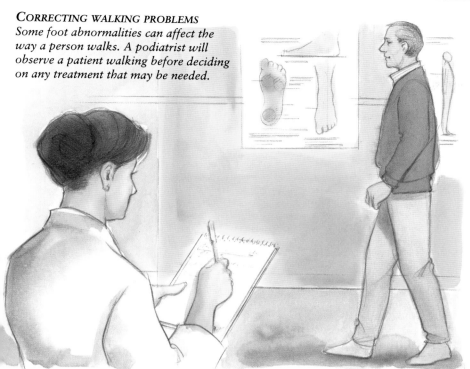

CORRECTING WALKING PROBLEMS
Some foot abnormalities can affect the
way a person walks. A podiatrist will
observe a patient walking before deciding
on any treatment that may be needed.

Where do podiatrists work?

Podiatrists work in private or group practices or clinics; hospitals and extended care facilities; municipal health departments and other public health services; and on faculties of schools in the health professions.

What training is required?

Practitioners must have completed a university degree and a four-year course of study at one of six accredited medical schools of podiatry in the United States. They must also have passed two board exams, one at the end of the second year of medical school and the other just prior to graduation.

For licensing, most states and Canadian provinces also require that candidates pass additional written and/or oral examinations and have completed at least one year of postgraduate residency training.

Some podiatrists do postgraduate training in nonsurgical areas that emphasize interdisciplinary, family, or orthopedic medicine. Others concentrate on the surgical techniques required to treat complex foot disorders, such as hammertoes and bunions.

How do I get podiatric treatment?

You can find a practitioner by looking in your local telephone directory under "podiatrist" or "chiropodist" or ask your family physician for a recommendation. You can also check the Internet for listings of practices in your region. Look for the letters DPM (Doctor of Podiatric Medicine) after the name to indicate that the podiatrist is fully qualified. In the United States the doctor should also belong to the American Podiatric Medical Association (APMA), which sponsors seminars and continuing education programs. The comparable organization in Canada is the Canadian Podiatric Medical Association, based in Toronto. You should check with Medicare or your HMO to find out if podiatric care is covered.

What can I expect during a first visit?

If the visit is a routine one, the podiatrist will examine your feet and carry out any remedial treatment that is appropriate. The doctor will take note of the way you stand and walk and ask about any mobility problems you may have. You will probably be given advice on how to care for your feet and prevent future problems.

In the case of a physical abnormality, an appropriate orthotic device—such as a specially designed insole for your shoes—may be fitted and subsequently monitored to make sure it gives the necessary correction.

Other conditions, such as athlete's foot, can be difficult to cure in the short term and may need a course of treatment over several visits. A podiatrist may also provide ointments and other preparations that you can apply at home.

WHAT YOU CAN DO AT HOME

Always dry your feet well after washing, especially between the toes. Remove rough skin with an emory board or pumice stone and apply moisturizer to prevent hard skin from developing. Cut your toe nails straight across and file off sharp corners. Wear flip-flops in public showers and changing rooms to avoid infection. You should also wear well-fitted shoes.

If you have a circulatory disorder, you should inspect your feet regularly. Cover any cuts and abrasions with sterile dressings and seek medical advice as soon as possible if you notice problems.

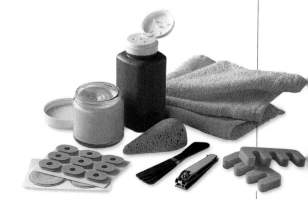

HOME FOOT CARE EQUIPMENT
Basic foot care items should include nail clippers, a pumice stone or file, talcum powder, moisturizing cream, and corn or callus pads if they are needed.

if they press against a nerve. Although you can gain some relief by bathing the foot in warm salt water or applying tea tree oil to the affected area, corns often need to be removed by a podiatrist or by treatment with medicated pads.

Bunions, which are a combination of thickening skin and bone growth around the joint of the big toe, generally form a lump at the side of the foot. Tight shoes must not be worn over bunions because pressure can cause the toe to bend inward. A podiatrist should be consulted; in very painful cases bunions may have to be removed by surgery.

Ingrown toenails are another common problem. They are often caused by incorrect nail cutting that forces the sides into the skin. Always cut your toenails straight across and file away any sharp edges.

RELIEVING ACHING FEET

You can relieve foot pain by rolling your foot over a rolling pin or unopened can of food. If your feet are stiff in the morning, rest them on a warm hot-water bottle or heating pad for 20 minutes. A foot soak at the end of a long day relieves tired feet, but you should not soak for more than 10 minutes.

REGULAR FOOT CARE AND MASSAGE

Tired and aching feet can cause a great deal of misery. Fortunately, feet respond well to a little care and attention. Taking 20 minutes once a week to give yourself a pedicure and a brief foot massage will revive your foot muscles and bones and put a spring in your step. If you regularly look after your feet, you are more likely to avoid such problems as ingrown toenails, hard skin, or circulation problems like chilblains. A home pedicure is very relaxing. Begin by soaking your feet for about 5 minutes.

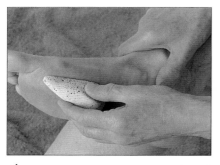

1 Use a pumice stone or emery board to smooth hard or rough skin on the heels and balls of the feet. Dry your feet carefully, paying particular attention to the skin between the toes.

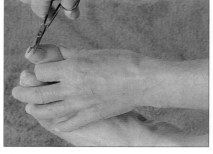

2 Trim your toenails straight across and use a file to remove any sharp points and edges. Pour moisturizer or massage oil onto your palm and massage well into the foot.

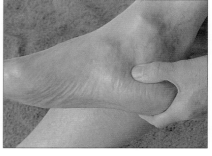

3 Make circular movements on your inner heel with your thumb, working from your instep to your ankle. Then squeeze upward along the tendon at the back of your ankles.

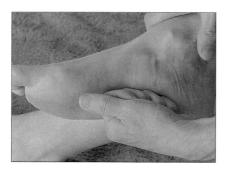

4 Hold your foot with one hand; make a loose fist with the other hand and make small circles on the soles of your feet with your knuckles. Continue this for a couple of minutes.

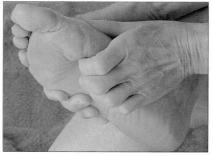

5 Hold the foot firmly with both hands so the heels of your hands touch each other on the top of the foot. Repeatedly press your fingers all over your sole.

CARE OF THE SKIN
Moisturize your feet and get rid of any hard skin by using a cornmeal scrub made with one tbsp of cornmeal mixed with 1 tsp of almond oil and 2 drops of peppermint essential oil.

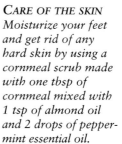

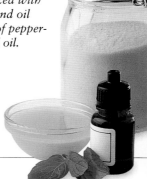

INDEX

—A—

Activities 45, 46, 47, 48
  and emotional benefit 45
  and holidays 48, 49
Acupuncture 132
Aerobic capacity 28
Aerobic exercise 104
Aging 16, 18, 19, 22, 26, 28, 29
  and blood pressure 56
  and bones 62, 65
  and cancer 74, 75, 76
  and cardiovascular system 54
  and diabetes 77
  and diet 19, 24, 80, 85, 88, 92
  and digestive system 60, 80
  and epilepsy 78
  and health screening 52, 53, 75
  and hearing 70
  and herbalism 19, 39, 57, 61
  and lifestyle 25
  and men's sexual health 67
  and muscles 63
  and occupation 25
  and physical changes 16, 27
  and physical health 16, 26
  and population 8, 33
  process of 25, 27
  and respiratory system 58
  and sight 71
  and smell 72
  and taste 72
  and touch 73
  and urinary system 66
  and volunteering 32
  and women's sexual health 68,
    69
Alcohol 81, 88, 91
  safe intake of 91
Alternative exercise 116
  Alexander technique 63, 116
  dancing 115, 116
  t'ai chi 116
  yoga 116
Alzheimer's disease 25, 77, 123
Anemia 57
Angina 55
Antiaging foods 85, 87
Antioxidants 19, 23, 74, 85, 86,
    88, 89
  and antiaging 23
  beta carotene 82, 89
  and cancer 85
  and cell protection 23
  flavonoids 86
  phytochemicals 85
  selenium 86, 87
  vitamin A 82, 86, 89
  vitamin C 82, 86, 89
  vitamin E 83, 86

zinc 84, 86
Apoptosis 18, 19, 23
Appetite 92, 102
Aqua aerobics 108
Arnica 116
Aromatherapy 111, 132
  essential oils 42, 132
Arthritis 30, 65, 90
  copper bracelets 65
  and exercising 109, 116
  gout 65
  osteoarthritis 65, 90
  rheumatoid arthritis 65, 90
Asthma 59
Atherosclerosis 57, 88

—B—

Bach, Dr. Edward 43
  flower remedies 43
Backache 30, 64
Bacteria 19, 98, 149
Balanced diet 80, 140
Baldness, cures 151
Bandler, Richard 120
Bardot, Brigitte 49
Basal metabolic rate (BMR) 27,
    28, 81, 102
Bates eye method 71
Bereavement 42, 43
  counselors 37
Biological age 17
Bioflavonoids 86
Biomarkers 17, 27, 28
  and aerobic capacity 28
  and blood pressure 28
  and cholesterol 28
  and metabolism 27, 28
  and muscle mass 27, 28
Blackman, Honor 27
Bladder 66, 69
Blood pressure 28, 56, 88
Body mass index (BMI) 139
Body shape 136, 137, 140
Body temperature 80
  regulation of 28
Bones 62
  density 28, 62
  fractures 62, 89
  osteoblasts 62
  osteoclasts 62
Brain 19, 27, 119, 122, 123
  and aging 119
  and Alzheimer's disease 25,
    123
  axons 119
  dendrites 119
  neurons 19
  structural plasticity of 119

synaptic gaps 119
  waves 130
Bras 138, 139
Bronchitis 59
Burns, George 8

—C—

Calcium 62, 63, 84, 89, 91
Calment, Jeanne 9
Calories 81
  and weight loss 140
Cancer 19, 23, 25, 74, 75, 89
  diet and 89
  and free radicals 23
  and preprogrammed cell death
    19
  risks for 76
  screenings for 75
  warning signs of 74
Candidiasis 68
Carbohydrates 81
Cardiovascular system 27, 54,
    55, 99
  chelation therapy 55
Caregivers 43
Carrot and lentil soup 92
Cells 18, 19, 22, 23
  accumulated damage theory
    19, 22
  advanced glycosylation end
    products 23
  behavior of 19
  DNA 19, 22, 84
  reproduction of 18, 19
Chang E 40
Chelation therapy 55
Chess 125
Children 40, 44
Chiropodist 154
Cholesterol 28, 54, 88
  high levels of 25, 88
  high-density lipoprotein
    (HDL) 28, 54
  low-density lipoprotein (LDL)
    28, 54
Chronological age 17
Cigarette smoking 22, 58
Circulation 54
  problems with 57
Clothes 136
  and colors 136
  and fit 136
Collagen 19, 141, 149, 153
Collagen implants 147
Colors 136, 137
Constipation 90
Container gardening 94
Coping skills 30

Cosmetic surgery 147
  collagen implants 147
  dermabrasion 147
Coughs, colds, and influenza 59
Counselors 36
Cystitis 67, 68

—D—

Daily calorie intake 81
Damiana 39
Dancing 115, 116
  line dancing 115
David, Elizabeth 88
Deafness 70
Death 18, 42
  bereavement 37, 42, 43
  bereavement counselors 37
Debt counselors 37
Degenerative problems 77
Dehydration 80
Dehydroepiandrosterone
    (DHEA) 19
Dental care 149
  crowns 150
  dental implants 150
  dentures 149, 150
  tooth whiteners 150
Depilatory cream 152
Depression 29, 30, 128
Dermatitis 144
Dermatologist 144–145
Diabetes 28, 77, 89
  blood sugar tolerance 28
  degenerative problems of 77
  hypoglycemia 89
  prevention 77
Diet 16, 22, 23, 27, 80, 82, 83,
    84, 88, 92
  and aging 80
  Chinese diets 25
  dietary reference values (DRV)
    80
  menopause diet 91
  recommended dietary
    allowance (RDA) 80
Digestion 60, 99
  constipation 90
  digestive enzymes 60
  diverticulosis 60
  hiatal hernia 60
  indigestion 60
Divorce 41

—E—

Ear infection 70
Eating habits 93
Echinacea 19
Einstein, Albert 119

Electrolysis 152
Emotions 27, 30, 32, 33, 36, 38,
    127, 132
    and aging 127, 132
    and bereavement 42, 43
    and change 27
    and retirement 33
Energy requirements 81
Epilepsy 78
Essential fatty acids 54, 82, 123
Essential oils 42, 132
Estrogen 19, 62, 88
    receptors 69
Evans, William 28
Exercise 16, 22, 27, 64, 98, 99,
    103, 104, 105
    aerobic 104
    and balance 99, 110
    benefits of 99
    and body temperature 104
    for flexibility 64, 103, 105
    and safety 107
    for strength 104
    non-weight-bearing
        64, 108
Eyeglasses 138

—F—

Facial massage 143
Family relationships 44
Fats 61 82
    and health 55
Feng shui 130
Fiber 81, 88
Financial planning 33, 35
Fitness assessment 114
Fluid intake 80
Flu relief 59
Food allergy 60
Food and hygiene 96
    safety 96
Foot care 153–156
    for aching feet 156
    for bunions 156
    for corns 153
    for fungal infections 153
    for ingrown toenails 156
    massage 156
Footwear 153
Fountain of youth 10, 80
Free radicals 19, 22, 23, 86
Friendship 44, 45, 46
Fruit fool 85
Funeral 43

—G—

Gardening 100
    garden jobs 101
    lifting technique 100
Garlic 55, 85, 87
General practitioner 20, 52
Genes 18, 22, 24
    bcl-2 gene 19, 23

genetic code 23
genetic inheritance 24, 25
    rescue gene 19, 23
    suicide genes 19
Genitourinary system 66–69
    cystitis 67, 68
    male problems 67
    and menopause 68–69
    urinary problems 66–68
    vaginal problems 68
Geriatrician 20–21
Gerontology 8, 20, 21, 24, 52
Ginkgo biloba 85, 87, 134
Ginseng 134
Glycosylation 23
Grandparents 28, 44
Green-lipped mussel 65
Gray power 47
Grief 29, 42
    counselor 29
Grinder, John 120
Growth hormone 22
Gum disease 150

—H—

Hair 151, 152
    style 152
    unwanted hair 152
Hair color 152
    graying 151
    herbal rinses 152
Hair loss 151
    and diet 151
    hairpieces 152
Happiness 44
Harman, Dr. Denham 19
Headaches, foot bath for 133
Health clubs 114
Health screening 52
Healthy diet 80, 85, 87
Hearing aids 70
Hearing loss 70
Heart function 54
Heart disease 54–56
    angina 55
    chelation therapy for 55
    risks for 54
Heat-shock genes 22
HeLa cells 9
Helpmann, Robert 12
Hemoglobin 57
Hemorrhoids 60
Herbs
    for cardiovascular health 55
    chamomile 142, 151
    damiana 39
    for digestive problems 61
    echinacea 19
    ginkgo biloba 85, 87, 134
    ginseng 134
    for health 93
    for memory 134
    rosemary 151
    sage 134

for taste 72, 93
    for varicose veins 57
High blood pressure
    (hypertension) 30, 56, 88
Hodgkin's disease 144
Homeopathy 111
Hormone replacement therapy
    (HRT) 64
Hormones 19, 22, 25
Hosak, Everitt 98
Hutton, Lauren 140
Hydrotherapy 133
Hypothermia 78

—I—

Immune system 22, 25, 30, 74,
    82, 83, 92
Impotence 67
Incontinence 66
Influenza vaccination 21
Intelligence 118
    crystallized 118
    fluid 118
Internet 122
Iron 56
Irritable bowel syndrome 30

—J—

Joints 64, 65, 99, 108, 112
    and arthritis 65, 112
    and exercise 108, 112
    synovial fluid in 62

—K—

Kegel exercises 69
Kidneys 27, 66
Kidney stones 66, 67
Kitchen garden 94

—L—

Labors of Hercules 114
Lactose intolerance 83
Lancashire hot pot 84
Laurel wreaths 134
Life expectancy 24, 25
Light therapy 128
Line dancing 115
Liver 27
Liver spots 145
Lobe stroking 131
Loneliness 40
Longevity 9, 19, 25, 26, 87
Lung diseases 58, 59
    emphysema 59
    pneumonia 59
Lungs 27, 58–59
    gas exchange 22
Lutein 91
Lymphocyte 25

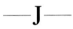

Macular degeneration 90, 91
Magnetic resonance imaging
    scan (MRI) 56
Massage 73, 132, 134, 143,
    151, 156
    and aromatherapy 132
    facial 143
    foot 134, 156
    scalp 151
    types of strokes 73
Menopause 68–69, 90, 91
    diet for 91
    male 67
    natural therapies for 68
    and osteoporosis 62, 63
    vitamins that benefit 69
Mind games 118
Mind over matter 112
Minerals 84
    selenium 86
    zinc 86
Mobility 99, 112
    and balance 99, 110
    and pain relief 112
Moisturizers 145, 146
Molecules 22, 86
Monounsaturated fat 88
Moving 49, 50
Muscle mass 28
Muscle tone 98
Muscles 27, 62, 99
    and exercise 99, 102, 104,
        106–108, 110–112, 115–116
Musculoskeletal system 62–65
Music 122

—N—

Neckache 30
Neuro-Linguistic Programming
    (NLP) 120, 121
Neurons 119
Neurotransmitters 119
Noradrenaline 128
Nutrients 80, 87

—O—

Oat fruit crumble 89
Obesity 88
Occupation 25
O'Keeffe, Georgia 47
Omega–3 fatty acids 86, 90,
    123
Osteoarthritis 65, 90
Osteoporosis 20, 62, 89, 90
Overhydration 81
Overweight 88, 139
Ozone layer 22
    and skin aging 22
    and free radicals 22

—P—

Parkinson's disease 20, 77
Pasteur, Louis 25
Pasteur Institute 21
Pectin 88
Pedicure 156
Pensions 35
  and inflation 35
Phobia 120
Phytochemicals 85
Pilates 63, 102
Pilates, Josef 102
Plaque 150
Podiatrist 153–154
Pollution 22, 24
Polyunsaturated fatty acids 82
Pool safety 109
Positive attitude 28, 44
Postmenopausal problems 69
Posture 62, 106, 138
Preretirement course 33
Programmed cell death 18, 19
  and chromosomes 18, 19, 22
Prostate problems 67
Protein 19, 23, 82
Pruritus 145
Psychological age 17
Psychoneuroimmunology (PNI)
  25
Pulse 105
  taking your own 105
  testing 55, 105

—Q—

Quindo 128

—R—

Recipes 81, 82, 84, 85, 89, 90,
  92, 95
  baked potato with tuna and
    coleslaw 82
  carrot and lentil soup 92
  fruit fool 85
  Lancashire hot pot 84
  oat fruit crumble 89
  rice with chicken, onions, and
    mushrooms 95
  salmon steak with pesto sauce
    90
  vegetable lasagna 81
Redundancy 32
Reflexology 134
Reishi mushroom 11
Relationship counselor 39
Relationships 36, 37
Relaxation techniques 30, 42
  for arthritis 24
  for arthritis pain 64, 65
  for baldness 151
  for cardiovascular problems
    54, 55, 56, 57, 134
  for colds and flu 59

for digestive problems 61
for ear infections 70
for eyestrain 71
for female genital problems 68
for foot pain 156
for grief 42, 43
for headaches 59, 133
for insomnia 43, 131
for joint pain 112
for menopausal symptoms
  69, 91
for muscular aches 63, 112
for prostate problems 67
for sexual problems 39
for wrinkles 19, 142
for yeast infections 61
Remarriage 41
Resistance training 28
Respiratory system 58–59
Retirement 28, 32, 33, 34, 35,
  36, 37, 44
  courses in 33
Retirement villages 49
Rice with chicken, onions, and
  mushrooms 95
Rosenberg, Irwin 28
Runting, Ernest 154

—S—

Safety rails 21
Salmon steak with pesto sauce
  90
Saturated fat 28, 82, 88
Scalp tonic 151
Seasonal colors 138
Sedentary lifestyle 25, 98
Selenium 86, 87
Self-confidence 30, 36
Self-defense 30
Self-fulfillment 50
Selye, Hans 30
Senses 70
Sensory memory 122
Sex life 99
  erections and 67
  and sex drive 39
  and sex hormones 19, 40
  and sexuality 39, 40
  therapist for 37
Shoes 153
Shou Lao 85
Sight 71
Sight problems 71, 90
  macular degeneration 90
  presbyopia 71
Sinan 118
Skin 99, 145
  dermis 141
  elastin fibers 141
  epidermis 141
Skin care 141–148
  alpha hydroxy acids (AHAs)
    147

for men 146
  products 143
Sleep 130–131
Smell 72
Smoking 74, 88, 92
Soy protein 19
Spices 93
Spine 62, 64
Sports 114
  cycling 114
  squash 114
  swimming 114, 116
  tennis 114
  walking 114
Stamina 99
Stomach 60
Storing food 94, 96
  freezer labels 96
Strength 28
Strength exercises 110
Stress 16, 22, 25, 30, 36, 56,
  99, 129
  anxiety 30, 129
Stretching exercises 64, 105
Stroke 25, 56
Stroke recovery 56
Sun protection factor (SPF) 142
Surgical (skin) treatments 147

—T—

T'ai chi 116
Tansy 10
Taoism 10, 11, 133
Target training zone 105
Taste 72
Tastebuds 72
Tea 85
Teeth 149–150
  correct care of 149
  dentures 150
  toothbrushes for 150
Telomeres 18, 19
Tendinitis 116
Testosterone 19, 39
Therapies 19, 28, 39, 42, 43, 44,
  57, 61, 63, 65, 67, 68, 73,
  111, 112, 116, 120, 121,
  128, 132, 133, 134, 143,
  151, 156
  Alexander technique 63, 116
  aromatherapy 43, 65, 111, 132
  Bach flower remedies 43
  herbalism 19, 39, 57, 61,
    67, 68
  hydrotherapy 133
  light therapy 128
  massage 73, 132, 134, 143,
    151, 156
  meditation 42
  Neuro-Linguistic Programming
    (NLP) 120, 121
  positive thinking 28, 44, 112
  quindo 128

reflexology 134
  t'ai chi 116
  transcutaneous nerve
    stimulation (TENS) 112
  visualization 42, 132
  yoga 63, 116
Thirst 80
Thymus gland 22
Tinnitus 70
Tithonus 17
Touch 73
  and massage 73, 132, 134
Toxins 19
Tranquilizers 129
Transcutaneous nerve
  stimulation (TENS) 112
Trans-fats 82
Treating injuries 110

—U—

Ultraviolet (UV) rays 142
Underweight 88, 139

—V—

Vacations 47, 49
Vaginal problems 69–69
Varicose veins 57
Vegetable lasagne 81
Violence 25
Viruses 19
Visualization 42, 132
Vitamin A 82, 86, 89
Vitamin B 83, 84, 125
Vitamin C 82, 86, 89
Vitamin D 63, 83
Vitamin E 83, 86
Vitamin K 83
Vitamins 82, 83, 86, 89
  fat-soluble 82
  for menopausal problems 69
  supplements 85
Volunteering 28, 32, 33, 46

—W—

Walking 28, 114
Walnuts 89
Warm-up exercises 106
Weight and appetite 102
Weight problems 27, 139–140
Wesley, Mary 35
Winfrey, Oprah 87
Wrinkles 19, 26, 136, 141

—Y—

Yeast infections 61
Yoga 113, 116

ACKNOWLEDGMENTS

Carroll & Brown Limited
would like to thank
Age Concern, The British Heart
Foundation, The British Library,
The Club House Day Centre,
Help the Aged

Editorial assistance
Richard Emerson, Joel Levy,
Nadia Silver

Design assistance
Rachel Goldsmith, Adelle Morris

DTP design
Elisa Merino

Photograph sources
8 (Top) King/Liaison/Frank
   Spooner Pictures
   (Bottom) Galleria Dell'
   Accademia, Venice/Bridgeman Art
   Library, London
9 (Top) Catherine Pouedras/
   Eurelias/SPL
   (Bottom) Dr Gopal Murti/SPL
10 Mary Evans Picture Library
11 Tony Stone Images
12 Reg Wilson
19 David Murray/C & B
20 Stockmarket
21 Mary Evans Picture Library
22 (Top) Prof K. Seldon & Dr T.
   Evans, Queen's University
   Belfast/SPL/DNA Molecule
   (Bottom) NOAA/SPL
23 Nancy Kedersha/SPL
24 (Left) Corbis – Bettmann
   (Right) Rex Features
25 Custom Medical Stock
   Photo/SPL
26 (Top) B. Gibbs/Trip
   (Bottom) K. Cardwell/Trip
27 Rex Features
30 Rex Features
32 R. Ian Lloyd/Hutchison Library
33 Ferdnand Ivaldi/Tony Stone Images
35 Mirror Syndication International

37 Trip
39 Ivan Polunis/Harry Smith
   Collection
40 C. M. Dixon
41 L. D. Gordon/Image Bank
44 Stockmarket
47 (Top) Sally & Richard Greenhill
   (Bottom) Evans & Amery
49 Rex Features
54 Science Photo Library
56 Department of Nuclear
   Medicine/Charing Cross
   Hospital/SPL
58 Biophoto Association/SPL
60 (Top) Susan Leavines/SPL
   (Bottom) National Medical Slide
   Bank
62 (Top) J. C. Revy/SPL
   (Bottom left, middle and right)
   J. C. Revy/SPL
65 (Bottom left) Dr P. Marazzi/SPL
   (Bottom right) Princess Margaret
   Rose Hospital/SPL
66 (Top) Mehau Kulyk/SPL
   (Bottom) National Medical Slide
   Bank
70 (Top) BSIP DuCloux/SPL
   (Bottom) P. C. Werth Ltd.
74 Custom Medical Stock Photo/SPL
75 (Top) Science Photo Library
   (Bottom) Michael Abbey/SPL
80 Bibliotheque Nationale, Paris/
   Topham Picturepoint/Bridgeman
   Art Library, London
84 Jim Holmes/Axiom
85 Board of Trustees: National
   Museums and Galleries on
   Merseyside (Lady Lever Art
   Gallery, Port Sunlight/Bridgeman
   Art Library, London)
87 (Top) Rex Features
   (Bottom) Holt Studio
   International
88 Jill Norman/David Bailey
94 Gilda Pacitti
98 News Team International
   Limited
100 Chris King/National Trust
    Photographic Library

102 Physicalmind Institute, Santa Fe,
    USA
112 David Russell/Garden Picture
    Library
114 AKG Photo, London
    (Bottom) Kaz Mori/Image Bank
115 S. Grant/Trip
116 Angela Hampton/Family Life
    Pictures
118 E. T. Archive
119 U.S. Library of Congress/SPL
120 *The Gestalt Journal Press*
123 Science Photo Library
125 Art Institute of Chicago/
    Bridgeman Art Library, London
127 John Walmsley
133 Eye Ubiquitous
134 Kunsthistorisches Museum,
    Vienna/Bridgeman Art Library,
    London
140 Rex Features
141 Valley of the Queens, Thebes,
    Egypt/Bridgeman Art Library,
    London
142 David Murray/C & B
152 Rex Features
154 J. C. Dagnall

Illustrators
Joanna Cameron, John Geary,
Sue Hellard, Sandie Hill,
Janice Nicolson, Josephine Sumner,
Anthea Whitworth, Paul Williams

Photographic assistants
Alex Hanson, Mark Langridge

Hair and make-up
Kim Menzies, Jess Owen

Picture research
Sandra Schneider

Research
Nadia Silver

Index
Denise Alexander

075–012–02